THE THERAPY OF THE WORD
in Classical Antiquity

THE THERAPY OF THE WORD
in Classical Antiquity

by Pedro Laín Entralgo

Edited and translated by
L. J. Rather and John M. Sharp

Yale University Press, New Haven and London, 1970

Copyright © 1970 by Yale University.
First published in Madrid, 1958, as *La Curación por la Palabra en la Antigüedad Clásica*
All rights reserved. This book may not be reproduced, in whole or in part, in any form (except by reviewers for the public press), without written permission from the publishers.

Library of Congress catalog card number: 72-99828
Standard book number: 300-01204-7
Designed by Marvin Howard Simmons,
set in Caledonia type,
and printed in the United States of America by Vail-Ballou Press, Inc., Binghamton, N.Y.

Distributed in Great Britain, Europe, Asia, and Africa by Yale University Press Ltd., London; in Canada by McGill-Queen's University Press, Montreal; and in Mexico by Centro Interamericano de Libros Académicos, Mexico City.

Contents

Foreword ix

Preface xvii

Prologue xxi

1. THE THERAPEUTIC WORD IN THE HOMERIC EPIC 1
   The Homeric epic in the mind of modern man
   I   Illness in the *Iliad* and the *Odyssey*. Origin and nature of illness.
   II The Homeric idea of Nature.
   III The cure of illness in the Homeric epic. Therapeutic purification. The magic charm. "Cheering speech."

2. FROM HOMER TO PLATO 32
   I   The culture of the Greek Archaic Age as a guilt-culture. Illness in the man of the Greek Archaic Age.
   II The therapeutic action of the word in the Greek lyric and tragic poets. The magic charm. Orphism. Dionysiac cult. The cult of Apollo. Mysteries of Eleusis. The therapeutic word in the temples of Asclepius. Metaphoric use of the terms *epôdê, thelktêrion,* and *kêlêma*. The goddess Persuasion. Psychological and therapeutic action of the persuasive word.
   III Therapy of the word in the pre-Socratic philosophers and in the Sophists. Historical significance of pre-Socratic philosophy. The pre-Socratic

philosophers and therapy of the word: Pythagoras, Empedocles, and Heraclitus. The Sophists. The Sophistic movement and verbal persuasion. Gorgias and Antiphon. Democritus and word therapy.

3. THE PLATONIC RATIONALIZATION OF THE CHARM   108
    I   The charm in Plato. Direct, metaphorical, and analogical use of the term *epôdê*.
    II   The curative charm of the *Charmides*. Healing and *sôphrosynê*. Rationalization of the charm. The Platonic theory of curing by the word. The Platonic idea of health.
    III Word therapy and purification of the soul.
    IV   Result of the inquiry.

4. THE WORD IN HIPPOCRATIC MEDICINE   139
Unity and diversity of the *Corpus Hippocraticum*.
    I   The novelty of Hippocratic thought. Nature of disease. Cause of disease. Treatment. Idea of *physis* (inborn, natural quality). Hippocratic medicine and the *logos* (word).
    II   The Hippocratic *logos* (word) as communicative language. The word as prayer, as question, as vehicle for a prescription, as prognostic judgment, as instrument of prestige, and as means of enlightenment.
    III The word of the Hippocratic physician as an agent of persuasion. The magic charm in the *Corpus Hippocraticum*. Hippocratic psychotherapy. Hippocratic psychosomatic pathology. Limitation of Hippocratic psychotherapy.

5. THE POWER OF THE WORD IN ARISTOTLE   171
Aristotle, heir and gainsayer of Plato.
    I   The *Rhetoric* of Aristotle and verbal psycho-

therapy. The character of the speaker. The frame of mind of the listener. What the orator says. Aristotelian psychology of verbal persuasion.

II The *Poetics* of Aristotle: tragic catharisis. The fundamental texts. Aesthetic, ethical, and medical interpretations. Bernays' medical interpretation. The recent contributions of Döring, J. Croissant, Kommerell, Dirlmeier, Schadewaldt, Flashar, and Pohlenz. Critical remarks.

III Tragic catharsis and the *logos* (word). Attic tragedy and Greek life. The "pleasure" of tragedy. The tragic situation. Theory of "the tragic." The tragic action. The internal order of tragic action. Qualities and course of tragic action. Affective aspect of the state of mind. Genesis and structure of tragic catharsis. Comparison of opinions.

Conclusion　　　　　　　　　　　　　　　　　240

  I   Historical summary.
  II Systematic summary.

Index of authors　　　　　　　　　　　　　　249

Foreword

Walter J. Ong

How the word relates to the rest of actuality has always been a major philosophical question. Indeed, like the question of the one and the many, or act and potency, or existence and essence, or yang and yin, or Apollo and Dionysus, or in our day being and time, it is one of those questions in terms of which all the other questions in philosophy can ultimately be framed.

The relationship between the word and the rest of actuality mystifies us deeply enough when it is taken in the abstract or perhaps in the framework of our own culture. In the framework of an earlier or an alien culture, the relationship becomes even more difficult to comprehend, for we soon find that attitudes toward the word in another culture are not necessarily our own.

The present work plunges the reader into ancient Greek culture at a point where it appears to us quite strange in its addiction to the word, and particularly to the spoken word. Dr. Laín Entralgo's Prologue singles out medicine as, in Vergil's words, one of the "silent arts" (*mutae artes*) whose practitioner is "without glory" (*inglorius*). This is clear evidence that one of the problems in classical antiquity as late as Vergil's time remained that of granting status to intellectual achievement remote from oral performance. The ancients were strongly verbomotor. By any standards generally operative in modern society the classical world was overcommitted to speech. Oratory enjoyed more prestige than did science.

At least since Freud the modern world has been aware of the potential in logotherapy and of the need to define its range —the possible effectiveness of the use of speech in restoring a person to health, as by vocalizing the contents of consciousness in free association, by dialogue between physician and patient, by interpretation of dreams or of other phenomena, and the like. But in classical antiquity the problem of discovering the proper role for the word in therapy was the reverse of that encountered when modern psychotherapy came into being, even though Freud's resort to models drawn from classical antiquity (most notably perhaps, the "Oedipus" complex) might suggest at first blush that the problem was the same. With Freud and those who have come after him (whether followers or pursuers) the problem has been to reestablish the effectiveness of verbal (generally oral) therapy in a milieu overreliant on the purely somatic. With the ancient Greeks, the problem was to sort out what might be truly therapeutic in the welter of verbal activities generated by a culture where both mores and academic education were dominantly rhetorical.

In the present learned and remarkably urgent book, Dr. Laín Entralgo traces the gradual refinement of the Greeks' ideas concerning the use of the word for therapy. Early attempts at logotherapy included crude magic but also the more acceptable "cheering speech" of Homer. This was superseded by the "apt words" which Plato recommends that physicians apply to their patients either to convince them (by dialectic) or to persuade them (by rhetoric), as may be necessary to produce in them the *sōphrosýnē* or tempered accord of everything in their being without which true health is not realized and physical medication ineffective. Plato was at this juncture concerned expressly with true verbal therapy. But he stopped here, as Dr. Laín Entralgo shows, at the level of conscious appeal and response. The poets he consequently found to be undesirables, for they stirred up violent emotions and thereby warred against the mind.

Accepting Plato's verbal therapy by conviction and persuasion as at times effective, Aristotle went further and carried his insight to the point where dialectic and rhetoric are transcended in tragedy. For Aristotle thought of tragedy as allied not only with religion but also with medicine. Tragic catharsis tempered the patient's constitution by releasing the violent

Foreword

emotions which Plato, less in tune with our present-day psychotherapy, wanted simply to suppress by outlawing tragedy. Aristotle recognized that when emotional charges build up, a good physician could indeed often work them out of his patient, as Plato wished, with strong argument or gentle persuasiveness. But emotions, particularly the deepest and most troublesome of them, could also be exorcized or "purged" by being brought to a state of tension which was suddenly resolved, as in tragedy, by means which were both "musical" (subconceptual) and rational as well in the insight they provided. Although the resolution was achieved not by entering directly into the real lifeworld but by entering into the world of "imitation" life, or art, nevertheless it had true medical, therapeutic value. Aristotle succeeded in defining simultaneously the grounds of a medical procedure and of aesthetic appeal, and probably without quite amalgamating them.

In doing so, he put new order into the relationship of the verbal to the nonverbal and thus served a great need for Greek culture. His solution remained, however, to a significant degree suspended in the verbomotor fabric of Greek thought, for it appears chiefly in his *Rhetoric* and *Poetics*, both concerned with the *artes sermocinales* or arts of discourse.

In the present work Dr. Laín Entralgo does not go into the larger question of the place of verbalization itself, and particularly oral verbalization, throughout classical culture. And for a very good reason: apart from the fact that his concern is specifically the use of verbalization for therapy, most of the significant work bearing on the larger question has been published since his present work appeared, in its original Spanish form, in 1958. It is a tribute to the erudition and intelligence of the author that the recent studies of primitive orality and of the shifts from an oral to a chirographic culture (and subsequently to a typographic and then an electronic culture) have not at all outmoded the present volume but have rather made it more urgent.

In fact, the appearance of this present work in English, in which most of the studies concerning the communications media shifts have thus far been done, is sure to suggest points of live contact between Dr. Laín Entralgo's findings and those of scholars and psychologists concerned with the more general characteristics of oral or nonliterate cultures, such as Milman Parry, Albert B. Lord, Eric A. Havelock, J. C. Carothers, Marvin Opler, and many others who can be found listed extensively in my own work, *The Presence of the Word*, and need not be relisted here.

The points of contact are established by our newly acute awareness of how oral classical antiquity was, despite its use of writing. Man has been in existence at least 500,000 years and without writing during almost all this entire span, for the first real scripts date from only around 3500 B.C. and the alphabet in its earliest form from only around 1500 B.C. The classical Greek world was only beginning to reconstitute within a chirographic economy the oral heritage of hundreds of thousands of years of human thought and expression quite free of any association with writing systems. Among the salient features of the earlier oral economy which were undergoing change in the era of which Dr. Laín Entralgo writes, three relate especially to his findings.

First, in a culture without writing, speech serves not only to express what is lodged in the mind, but in its various stylized configurations—its themes, formulas, proverbs, epithets, and the like—also to store and retrieve verbalized knowledge. Without the storage systems which writing later provides, knowledge has to be constantly regurgitated and uttered ("out-ered") or it simply disappears. Speech has to be given special patterns of a mnemonic sort, for man knows only what he can recall, and the only resource for verbal recall in an oral culture is memory. Nothing can be "looked" up (with the eye); everything must be "called" up or "recalled" (retrieved by voice and ear). Speech patterns are crucial. For this reason, even in the most laconic early cultures, utterance is attended to and valued in ways it will seldom be once writing takes hold.

Secondly, an oral noetic economy tends to connect all knowledge, even the most abstract, more or less directly with the human lifeworld and in this way limits abstraction. For, as Havelock has shown in his *Preface to Plato* (1963), even the equivalent of what we today isolate as scientific knowledge, what we today preserve through writing or print or computers in "objective" mental enclaves as sciences or disciplines or merely "information" apart from the push and pull of human life, is in an oral culture closely associated with the world of human action and interaction. What we encapsulate in demographic lists (city or national directories) or trade manuals is found, in its nearest approximations, largely in the narratives of oral cultures, which are unable to constitute knowledge in elaborately categorized form. Thus the list of ships, leaders, and followers in the *Iliad* ii.494–875, or the account of shipbuilding in the *Odyssey* v.225–61. In an oral culture where else than in performing a lengthy narrative would an occasion offer itself to utter aloud this amount of material regarding population or shipbuilding?

As a result of this close association of the equivalent of "science" with what we have called the push and pull of human life, in oral cultures the role of the orator, the skilled rhetorician or public speaker who gives direction to human activity, is overcharged by our present-day standards. In being concerned with human action, he is caught up with everything. It is under these circumstances that the Sophists, essentially public speakers and trainers of public speakers, can profess to be masters of all knowledge, and that Cicero in his writings on oratory can maintain that the orator must be master of everything that men know.

Thirdly, and finally, in an oral culture, which knows words only in their natural habitat, that is, the world of sound, words necessarily carry with them a special sense of power. For sound always indicates the present use of power. A primitive hunter can see a buffalo, smell a buffalo, touch a buffalo, and taste a buffalo when the buffalo is dead and motionless. If he *hears* a buffalo, he had better watch out: something is going on. No other sensory field has this dynamism which marks the field of sound. So long as words are known only directly and without interference for what they ultimately are—sounds—and cannot possibly be imagined to be what they really are not—marks on a surface—they are sensed as physically powered events, happenings, of a piece with all present actuality. The effects of this direct way of conceiving of words—Homer's "winged words," both fleeting and powerful—are too manifold and massive to discuss here. But it should be noted that a feeling for words as primarily spoken—which lingered with diminishing vigor even after the invention of print—complicates the question whether the power which primitive peoples sense in words can be reduced simply to magic.

Such are some of the general features of the orality out of which Greek culture was working at the time when questions concerning the therapy of the word arose. Havelock has shown in great detail that precisely in Plato's lifetime Greek culture was completing its move from orality through craft literacy (when you hired a man to write a letter as you hired a man to build a boat) to the stage where, finally "the cultivated Greek public had become a community of readers" (p. 41), even though by our standards they remained incredibly oral still. Writing was affecting the storage of knowledge. The possibility of lists and of "looking up" what others had set down in nonmnemonic form was opening new horizons for abstract thought. It was becoming possible to compose and to think the way Plato does in the *Republic*.

In the light of Havelock's findings, Plato's rejection of the poets and his touting of his "ideas" appear as two sides of the same coin. In both cases Plato was showing his dissatisfaction with the old verbomotor *paideía* and noetic activity which limited thought patterns to those which could be stored and retrieved orally. The kinds of knowledge storage and retrieval which writing had finally made possible also made it possible to free thought from utter reliance on epithets, formulas, clichés, and "sayings" of all sorts, and from inevitable involvement in the human lifeworld, and to develop dispassionate, thoroughly abstract thinking of the sort represented by the world of Platonic "ideas," which were fixed, "pure," uninvolved with the push and pull of human living. In the Seventh Letter and in the *Phaedrus* (274), it is true, Plato expressly favors oral, living speech over the dead fixity of writing, but the general drive of his thought in fact rejects the old noetic economy in favor of one which only writing made possible. And in outlawing the poets from his *Republic* he shows his hand by overprescribing.

Aristotle's clarification of the role of the word in therapy is evidently a part of this movement of Greek thought from an oral noetic economy to the more "scientific" or abstract economy of carefully worked out causality which writing makes possible. And the failure of subsequent ancient medicine to take up Aristotle's lead probably attests the persistence of oral modes of thought. The present work points out that for post-Aristotelian medicine any therapy of the word was simply an attempt at magic. Connections of magic with orality have been suggested here above.

Dr. Laín Entralgo's work combined with that of Havelock shows that Aristotle, however, rejects the old oral world less totally than does Plato, despite the latter's protestation of love for the spoken word. Just as in the *Rhetoric* Aristotle made persuasion an honest woman subject to the abstract *theōría* of a systematic *téchnē* which writing made possible without demanding of her the total rationality which the emergent chirographic culture was beginning to canonize and which Plato favored, so in his doctrine of logotherapy Aristotle is less rationalist than Plato. Plato had admitted verbal therapy only at the conscious levels reached in rational conviction and persuasion. Aristotle acknowledged this kind of therapy, but added the therapy of *kátharsis*, which was to a degree effected by conscious, intense insight into the human situation but also by factors less articulate, more "musical."

The foregoing remarks have not exhausted the implications of Dr. Laín Entralgo's work, for his material and his learning are vast, and his arguments wide-ranging and always carefully nuanced. These particular implications are pointed out here to show some of the continuing large-scale relevance of this study completed over a decade ago in Spanish.

Perhaps they suggest even further relevance for the future as today the world moves in the new orality of our electronic era, where the telephone, loudspeaker, radio, and television give voice a new kind of currency. Our new secondary orality makes us in significant ways like those who lived in the old primary oral culture, although in equally significant ways it makes us vastly different, for it is derived orality, dependent on script and print. In our present circumstances we can lean, with Dr. Laín Entralgo, to Aristotle's tolerance rather than to Plato's alarmism. The chirographic culture which had grown up around Plato was making him suspicious of the old primary oral ethos. Trained in a chirographic and typographic ethos, many persons today are suspicious of the new secondary orality which beats in on our ears, and indeed thoroughly alarmed. We might follow Aristotle's discrimination, identifying as far as we can and accepting what is good and true and beautiful in orality, and rejecting only what is clearly not. Dr. Laín Entralgo's book has the true relevance and prescience here that we have learned to expect from studies treating the past as it should be treated, from the inside, within its own frame of reference, with a full command of the language and thought of the period and an intimate and sympathetic familiarity with the lifeworld of the time. Studies such as this have sure relevance for our day and for the future, especially when they are concerned with making clear how much of human experience and knowledge and love gathers around and in the word.

Saint Louis University

Preface

Dr. Pedro Laín Entralgo holds the chair in the history of medicine at the University of Madrid. Only one of his many books has hitherto appeared in English (*Mind and Body*, New York: P. J. Kennedy and Sons, 1956).* The work now being offered to the reader in translation is of very broad scope. It embraces all aspects of the therapeutic "power of the word," as that power was understood by physicians, philosophers, poets, and dramatists of ancient Greece, from Homer through Hippocrates, Plato, and Aristotle. In the course of his survey Laín Entralgo manages to take into account much of the pertinent literature contributed by recent German, French, and English scholars, as well as by those writing in his native Spanish. The translation was undertaken with the belief that the result would be of interest to general readers as well as to physicians, philosophers, intellectual historians, and other specialists.

The central topic of this book is the origin of a dominant trait of Western medicine, namely its strongly somatic orientation. Throughout most of its long history Western medicine has, so to speak, denied the power of the word in the treatment of human illness and put its faith in treatment by diet, drugs, and surgery. That dominant trait had its origin in the naturalistic medicine of classical Greece, roughly speaking in the fifth century B.C. Laín Entralgo first shows how healers in preclassical Greece employed the therapeutic power of the word. Their use of charms, prayers, and incantations, either alone or in conjunction with other forms of treatment, was in fact much like that met with in so-called primitive societies generally. The outlines of Greek natural science then became discernible, and in the fifth century Hippocratic medicine appeared on the scene. Hippocratic medicine was rationalistic, naturalistic, and scientific, whatever we may now think of its theories and their factual basis. But to achieve its scientific naturalism Hippocratic medicine had first to reject the old verbal therapy in the form that Laín Entralgo calls the "pre-rational." Medicine in the hands of the Hippocratic physicians became the "mute art," as Virgil was later to call it. Acts, not empty words, were required of the physician in the treatment of human illness. The object of naturalistic medicine was the human body, and the means to be employed were diet, drugs, and surgery. Successful treatment, according to the Hippocratic physicians, necessitated an understanding of the nature (*physis*) of the body (*sôma*). Their concern was not with divine or daemonic powers or, for that matter, with the soul (*psyché*) of the patient.

Was a flaw already discernible in the otherwise well-laid foundations of Greek medicine as early as the fifth century B.C.? It would seem so. For in the *Charmides* of Plato the physicians of Greece are said to be wanting in an appreciation of the significance of the whole and deficient, in consequence, in the management of those ailments brought on the body by the soul. Plato put these words into the mouth of a Thracian physician, and they should not be taken to represent his opinion in its entirety. Indeed, elsewhere in the *Dialogues* he seems to regard the medicine of his day as an exemplary art or technique. However that may be, Plato did develop what Laín Entralgo maintains may fairly be called a scientific technique of verbal psychotherapy, crowning the efforts in the same direction made by Sophists such as Gorgias. The historical irony of the situation is striking. At the very time that "pre-rational" verbal therapy was being discarded by the naturalistic physicians of the Hippocratic school the philosophers were successfully "rationalizing" verbal therapy. Thereby the Greek physicians might have learned to address themselves properly to the *psyché* of man, with words, as well as to his *sôma*, with diet, drugs, and surgery. But they did not, and in consequence the development of Western medicine went somewhat askew. Laín Entralgo remarks that it is as if the

Greek physicians had tacitly accepted Plato's proposal (made in the *Phaedrus*) to assign medicine the task of curing the body and to assign rhetoric, i.e. philosophy, the task of curing the soul. This division of labor can be found several centuries later in Cicero, for whom philosophy is *medicina mentis,* the medicine of the mind or soul.

As Laín Entralgo points out, it cannot be denied that the Hippocratic physicians were acquainted with the far-reaching changes in the body that might be produced by emotional disturbances. Yet even when they were aware of the emotional factors in a bodily ailment their treatment, insofar as it was "scientific," was purely somatic. Although they knew that words could and should be used on occasion to exhort or cheer their patients, they had no technique of verbal therapy. The soul could be altered by the proper use of food, drink, exercise, and baths, as the Hippocratic treatise *On Diet* states, and seemingly this was enough for the naturalistic physicians. Moving somewhat beyond the period covered by Laín Entralgo in this book, we find Galen in the second century of our era classifying disturbances of the emotions (*psychês pathê*) as one of six sets of factors causative of disease. We can even hear an echo of the *Charmides* in a remark by Galen that physicians in general paid too little attention to the role of the *psychê* as a cause of bodily ills, a remark made in connection with the illness of a woman that had baffled the physicians called in before him. But it seems that Galen himself had no technique of verbal psychotherapy with which to proceed once he had so skilfully laid bare the emotional roots of her ailment. And the medical historian can point to a succession of physicians who recognized, in the centuries thereafter, the influence of emotional disturbances on the health of their patients but used to a limited extent, if at all, means of therapy other than the traditional diet, drugs, and surgery.

The point is worth additional emphasis: Western physicians recognized clearly and explicitly that disturbances of the mind or soul could and did cause all manner of bodily disturbances, either alone or in conjunction with other factors, but they held that their business was to treat the body. The mind or soul was not within their province. And as far as the education of physicians is concerned, the canon of medical studies that became established in the universities of Europe was essentially that laid down by Galen, who himself relied mainly on Hippocratic sources. The Galenical canon had made its way to Europe via the Arabic writers and was then embodied in systematic treatises covering the whole of medicine. Using the modern terminology introduced by Fernel in the sixteenth century, the canon of medical studies included physiology (with the necessary anatomy and "chemistry"), pathology, hygiene, and therapy. Until the introduction of psychiatry into the medical curriculum a few generations ago it remained in principle unchanged.

A few remarks on the translation may be worth making here. I found myself unable to accomplish it alone and was fortunate enough to enlist the aid of Professor John M. Sharp. Regrettably we were unable to verify all of the citations in the text or furnish alternative editions where desirable. Nor could we in all cases retranslate from the original languages such passages as Laín Entralgo had translated into Spanish. Some of the citations have been verified and a few corrected, however, and we hope that our more scholarly readers will be indulgent. Valuable assistance in reviewing the final typescript and page proofs was given by Dr. John B. Frerichs. Mrs. Anne Wilde and her staff at the Yale University Press have been very helpful throughout. At Mrs. Wilde's suggestion Father Ong was invited to contribute a foreword.

L. J. RATHER

---

* ADDENDUM IN PROOF: Laín Entralgo's *Doctor and Patient* was issued in a paperbound edition in English in 1969.

Prologue

In the twelfth book of the *Aeneid*, the reader will find a curiously worded description of the medical art. Aeneas, seriously wounded, is about to receive expert help. To this task Iapix earnestly applies himself, a man who in order to prolong the days of his father, and in preference to other possible gifts of his protector Apollo, "chose knowledge of the power of herbs and ways of curing and to practice without glory the silent arts,"

> scire potestatem herbarum, usumque medendi
> maluit, et mutas agitare inglorius artes
> (*Aeneid*, XII, 396–97).

Faithful to this Vergilian characterization of his preference, Iapix, without words and with only his hands and his herbs, seeks in vain to cure Aeneas until Venus is moved to lend invisible and decisive aid.

Medicine is called *muta ars*, "the silent art." What meaning does this adjective have in Vergil's mind as a designation for medicine? Is its only purpose to emphasize the contrast between the ability chosen by Iapix and the higher-sounding talents Apollo had offered him with it: the cithara and the gift of prophecy? Or is the poet alluding at the same time to the vigor with which professional Greek and Roman medicine had forbidden the use of charms and musical spells? This we cannot ascertain. But perhaps the poetic expression in the *Aeneid* is not foreign to the view that was to appear four centuries later in the *Mulomedicina* of Vegetius: "Animals and men must not be treated with vain words but by the sure art of medicine";[1] or the explicit opinion of Soranus, recorded by

1. *Animalia et homines non inanibus verbis, sed certa medenti arte curentur.* Ernst Lommatzsch, ed. (Leipzig, 1903), p. 199, 3–4.

Prologue

Caelius Aurelianus: "They boast foolishly and vainly who believe that the power of an illness can be expelled with songs and chants." [2]

In contrast to superstitious and popular medicine, technical or scientific medicine must be a *muta ars,* an art without words. The difference between this way of viewing therapy, and modern practice, to which verbal psychotherapy is so essentially and inseparably bound, cannot be more obvious. The ancient physician did not know how nor did he wish to use language as a therapeutic device: such, at least, appears to be the conclusion forced on us.

But was this true of *all* medicine in classical antiquity? And to the extent that it does apply to ancient medicine, could the situation have been otherwise? If ancient literature is viewed from the intellectual position in which the medical historian of the twentieth century necessarily finds himself, and in the pure order of therapeutic action, does it contain any evidence of a *verbum* not as *inane* as that so roundly excoriated by Soranus and Vegetius? The following pages seek to answer these questions and at the same time to make a contribution to the history of the still not yet firmly established doctrine of verbal psychotherapy.

Pedro Laín Entralgo

Madrid, 1958

2. *Sed Sorani iudicio videntur hi mentis vanitate iactari, qui modulis et cantilena passionis robur excludi posse crediderunt.* Caelius Aurelianus, *De morbis acutis et chronicis,* J. Cr. Amman, ed. (Amsterdam, 1709), p. 555.

Chapter 1

The Therapeutic Word in the Homeric Epic

In the interpretation of the Homeric epic—and indeed of all Hellenic literature—a historian is exposed to two opposite dangers: one we shall call "idealization," and the other "primitivization."

From antiquity down to the nineteenth century, the *Iliad* and the *Odyssey* have always been both prototype and point of departure. The nostalgic eyes of historians, writers, and philologists have seen in them not only a model for literary creation but also the seed of almost everything in human affairs since: the good in the opinion of the majority; the bad, or at least part of the bad, in the judgment of some who are dominated by the illustrious spirit of Plato. For twenty-five centuries the Homeric poems have constituted the most genuine and outstanding example of a "classical" work. Whether with or without personal genius, in the presence of Homer all Western men have been the fellows of those *graeculi* recently studied so carefully by Félix Buffière.[1] Homer is the father or the grandfather of the West.

This view of the Homeric epic has never lost its vigor. Under its influence, perhaps unwittingly, are those who from time to time have taken up the problem of what is *not* to be found in the *Iliad* and the *Odyssey* in contrast to the usual consideration of what *is*.[2] But the fact is that since the nineteenth century, aided by the genetic and historical attitude

---

1. F. Buffière: *Les mythes d'Homère et la pensée grecque* (Paris, 1956).
2. This statement applies to authors who, spiritually established in the Christian conception of religion, have attributed to these poems an almost total lack of religion. "There never was a less religious poem than the Iliad," writes P. Mazon (*Introduction à l'Iliade*, Paris, 1948, p. 294); the so-called Homeric religion was "really anything but a

that appeared and established itself at that time, the historian and the philologist have begun to discern in those two famous poems not so much what was "origin" as what is "result." Without ceasing, of course, to be "classical" creations, the *Iliad* and the *Odyssey* have begun to reveal themselves as archaic documents. This, indeed, is the real significance of the famous Homeric problem; this innovation became even more evident when a glimpse was caught of the historic significance of the Greek epic by means of the techniques and discoveries of ethnology, as recently achieved by Nilsson, Dodds, Onians, and Moulinier.[3] To the shocked astonishment of the idealizing enthusiasm of the old Hellenists, the revered contents of Homer's hexameters are now being dissolved into "primitive" or "savage" ways of thinking and acting. The content is viewed not so much from the standpoint of what followed as from what may have preceded it. In other words: as a modern man, the Hellenist has regarded the classical as primitive and—at the same time—has converted the primitive into the classical. After all, the classics themselves had already said: *humani nihil a me alienum puto*.

After the systematic idealization of the Homeric work, the danger today is perhaps beginning to be an excessive primitivization. The ethnological study of the *Iliad* and the *Odyssey*, so fruitful, thought-stimulating, and refreshing, must not obscure sight of what Greek culture later became, and if both poems are comparable to the legends of the Bushmen and the Yakuts they are from a historical and human point of view also a great deal more than all of these. And as an archaic document both poems represent, one should not forget, the foundation of Western culture.

It is indeed true that this word of caution can hardly apply to the limited field with which I am dealing: the history of

---

religion," G. Murray had said previously (*Rise of the Greek Epic*, 4th ed. p. 265; quoted by E. R. Dodds in *The Greeks and the Irrational*, Berkeley and Los Angeles, 1951).

3. M. P. Nilsson, *Geschichte der griechischen Religion I* (Munich, 1941); E. R. Dodds; R. B. Onians, *The Origins of European Thought* (Cambridge, 1954); L. Moulinier, *Le pur et l'impur dans la pensée des Grecs d'Homère à Aristote* (Paris, 1952).

medical knowledge. Physicians studying Homer have in general fallen victim to the first of the two dangers mentioned above, victims both naive and enthusiastic. Moved by the ardor of their *Hellenophilia,* they have been accustomed to idealize the figure of the great Ionic poet to the point of converting him (as Galen said of Hippocrates) into "the discoverer of all good things." Take, for instance, the cleansing of the room in which Ulysses dealt savage and furious death to Penelope's suitors (*Od.,* XXII, 481–94). Once the bloodstains had been washed away, Ulysses "fumigated" with the smoke of burning sulfur (*theeion*) the murder chamber, the remaining rooms of the palace, and the courtyard. What is the meaning of this act? For O. Körner, the matter is obvious: it is a hygienic measure. The fact that Ulysses calls sulfur *kakôn akos,* a remedy of ills, would seem to prove this; those "ills" are necessarily diseases, Körner declares, since the *Odyssey* itself elsewhere calls physicians *iêtêres kakôn* (XVII, 384).[4] A. Botto is of the same opinion. To "disinfect" his house, writes the Italian physician, Ulysses "uses a most perfectly hygienic procedure," fumigation with sulfur. And he adds, "This system of disinfecting with sulfur, once used in Homer's times, has remained unchanged across the centuries, for it is still practiced in such cases.[5] But to discover that it was current at that time is rather surprising, just as the foresight governed by the most scrupulous hygienic policy and present in all these activities is also a subject for wonder." [6] According to all this, Homer must have been a farsighted predecessor of Guyton de Morveau and von Pettenkofer.

It is clear that Körner and Botto are medically idealizing the figure of the great Ionic bard. The former, devoted reader of the *Iliad* and the *Odyssey* though he is, forgets that the expression *kakon eidos* does not imply "diseased appearance" but rather "ugliness" (*Il.,* X, 316), and that *kakê gynê* means "evil

4. *Die aerztlichen Kenntnisse in Ilias und Odyssee* (Munich, 1929), p. 61.
5. A comment: Where and when did Botto have the opportunity to observe that a room in which a murder has been committed is fumigated with sulfur?
6. *Omero medico* (Viterbo, 1930), p. 161.

woman" and not "sick woman" (*Od.*, XI, 384). And both he and Botto—like many others, for these two interpreters are not alone—fail to recall that fumigation by the fumes of sulfur (*peritheiôsis*) was for many centuries in Greece a purifying or cathartic rite, a religious expedient against moral impurity rather than a hygienic measure in the modern sense of the word.[7]

In these reflections regarding the Homeric concept of human illness and its treatment, I hope to steer clear of both reefs. I shall of course emphasize insofar as necessary the archaic character of the epic, but without ignoring the perennially human and exemplary value that many of its pages possess. What sensitive-minded Western reader does not feel today, as was felt centuries ago, a delicate aesthetic and moral emotion as he relives within himself the parting of Hector and Andromache? And what man of science does not experience a deep and keen intellectual thrill upon reading in the *Odyssey* the reduction of the *physis,* the nature, of the *môly*—that mysterious plant so named by the gods—to a precise, clear, and verifiable set of visual properties? But this should not be an obstacle to an unglossed recognition of the archaic and in no sense "rational" character of the Homeric attitude toward the state of mind called *atê* in the epic, that rash blinding fury of the human soul, and toward so many other cosmic or psychological realities.

Faithful to this indispensable and promising middle way—which in an Aristotelian sense I shall endeavor to convert into the best way—I shall study in turn the Homeric idea of illness and medical treatment and the role played by the spoken word in the latter.

I. A detailed examination of the passages in which human illness appears in the epic enables us to distinguish four different ways of conceiving of and interpreting illness: the traumatic, the punitive, the environmental, and the demonic.

---

7. An eloquent passage from Plato in the *Cratylus* (406b) is sufficient to convince one of this. I do not understand how Moulinier, in his excellent book previously cited, can question the cathartic nature of this fumigation of Ulysses' palace. Could this burning of sulfur possibly have any other meaning?

It is evident that traumatic lesions are the affections most frequently mentioned in the *Iliad* and the *Odyssey*, particularly in the former, and most frequently commented upon by historians since Malgaigne's initial study.[8] No less than 172 are indicated and described in the two poems taken together, according to the painstaking calculations of Frölich and Botto. But for our purpose the wounding action of spears, swords, arrows, and stones near Troy or in the palace of Ithaca is less important than Homer's mental attitude toward this action. All of these affections have from the bard's point of view a common trait: all are the immediate results of an act of material violence, visible to the eyes of the spectator and rationally comprehensible to his mind. Let us recall the adventure of the Cyclops. Ulysses, who has shrewdly given his name as "No man," has just blinded the eye of Polyphemus. The latter cries out in the night and the Cyclops ask him from afar whether someone is slaying him by guile or by force. Polyphemus replies, "Noman is slaying me by guile, nor at all by force." To this the Cyclops answer, "If then no man is violently handling thee in thy solitude, it can in no wise be that thou shouldst escape the sickness sent thee by mighty Zeus. Nay, pray thou to thy father Poseidon, lord of the seas" * (*Od.*, IX, 406–12).

8. *Études sur l'anatomie et la physiologie de Homère* (Paris, 1842). The most important works on Homeric medicine—besides those of Körner and Botto previously mentioned—are the following: J. R. Friedrich, *Die Realien in der Iliade und Odyssee* (Erlangen, 1851); Ch. Daremberg, *La médecine dans Homère* (Paris, 1865); E. Buchholz, *Die homerischen Realien II, Erste Abtheil.* (Leipzig, 1881); H. F. Frölich, *Die Militärmedizin Homers* (Stuttgart, 1879); O. Schmiedeberg, *Über die Pharmaka in der Ilias und Odyssee* (Strasbourg, 1918); B. Coglievina, *Die homerische Medizin* (Graz, 1922). I have not thought it pertinent to set forth here, even in outline, the famous and endless "Homeric question." Anyone wishing to familiarize himself with the bibliography on the current state of the matter should read *Die Homerforschung in der Gegenwart* (Vienna, 1952), by A. Lesky, and the *Geschichte der griechischen Literatur* (Bern, 1957–58), by the same author. For my personal research I have considered the Homeric epic in its entirety as an expression of the most archaic mentality of the Greek people; according to the best qualified philologists of today (see, for example, W. Jaeger's opinion in his *Paideia*), this is entirely valid.

* Translation of the Homeric quotes here is taken with occasional modifications from the Lang, Leaf, Butcher, and Myers prose translation, Modern Library.

The first term of the Cyclops' dilemma—either illness resulting from external violence (*bia, biêphi*), or illness (*nousos*) sent by Zeus—obviously includes all pathological states the cause of which may be clearly seen and understood by the eye of a human being or a Cyclops, that is, traumatic lesions of any type.[9] Let us bear in mind Homer's precise nosological and etiological dichotomy.

Clearly distinguished from the traumatic affections, and even opposite to them, are the illnesses, so often fatal, visited by the gods upon men. The *Iliad* begins with the description of one such ailment: the plague inflicted by Apollo upon the Achaeans in punishment of Agamemnon's abduction of the daughter of Chryses (I, 8 ff). The punitive nature of the disease is here quite unquestionable. Such a view of a morbid accident also clearly appears in the case of the death of Niobe's twelve children. Niobe dared to compare herself to the goddess Leto, thus committing the sin of *hybris*, or excess, and was condemned to suffer the wrath of Apollo and Artemis, Leto's offspring, against her children: Apollo's arrows mortally wounded the six males, and those of Artemis the six females (*Il.*, XXIV, 605–06). The ailment from which the Cyclops thinks Polyphemus is suffering (in the previously cited passage) is on the other hand not attributed to divine punishment, even though sent by the gods; nor are the diseases that cause the death of Laodamia, mother of Bellerophon (*Il.*, VI, 205), nor of Andromachê's mother (*Il.*, VI, 428), nor of Rexenor (*Od.*, VII, 63), nor of the inhabitants of that Syrian isle where no one knows hunger and men die at an advanced age (*Od.*, XV, 403–11); neither does it appear probable that the doughty Bellerophon's melancholy—caused by the obstinate hatred of the gods, according to the Homeric text—is a punishment of

9. The second term of that dilemma—illness (*nousos*) sent by Zeus—probably referred, according to Dodds (p. 67) to a mental illness. The reasoning of the Cyclops who hears Polyphemus' lamentations was doubtlessly: if no man is wounding Polyphemus, Polyphemus is the victim of a distressing ailment of sudden, invisible, and, therefore, divine origin. For Homer madness is not the only ailment set by the gods (see my remarks on this subject in the following paragraph).

any transgression against divinity (*Il.*, VI, 200-01). The terrifying human problem of undeserved suffering is hinted at in these illnesses inflicted on mortals by the arrows of Apollo and Artemis.[10]

In other cases a natural cause, external and not traumatic, seems to be ascribed to illness: it is exemplified by the type of sickness above called "environmental." Ulysses alludes to this when he arrives naked on the Phaeacian shore and fears that he will die a victim of the night cold (*Od.*, V, 451 ff), and this, too, is what Hector seeks to avoid when, mindful of the possible harmful effect of the wine, he refuses the drink offered him by his mother (*Il.*, VI, 264-65), and what can be produced by the "deadly drugs" (*thymophthora pharmaka*) that Telemachus is to seek in Ephyra (*Od.*, II, 329). Less clear is the morbid, febrile character of the "excessive warmth" (*pollon pyreton*) caused by the constellation Orion, according to a disputed verse in the *Iliad*.[11]

10. Elsewhere (*Introducción histórica al estudio de la patología psicosomática*, Madrid, 1940), I have sought to give a historical and psychological interpretation to the idea of illness as a punishment of man by the gods. Evidence in support of such an idea appears in the societies forming the cultural level called "higher primitive culture" by ethnologists of the *kulturhistorische Schule*, and adopting various forms this concept continues to exist in the archaic Semitic and Indo-European cultures: more "personally" oriented in the former and more "naturalistically" in the latter. Everyone knows that the misfortune—or, if you will, the undeserved punishment—of the just man is to be one of the cardinal themes of Attic tragedy.

11. The poem reads: "blazing as the star that cometh forth at the end of summer—the *Opôra*—and plain seen his rays blaze forth amid the host of stars in the darkness of night, the star whose name men call Orion's Dog. Brightest of all is he, yet for an evil sign is he set, for he bringeth excessive heat to hapless mortals" (*Il.*, XXII, 25-31). Does the expression, "excessive heat," refer to fever? Brendel thought so as early as 1700, and so do Finsler, Coglievina, and Körner. "Sirius' appearance in the skies in the *Opôra* (August and September)," the latter writes, "coincides with the outbreak of malaria . . . Daremberg scoffs at Brendel's explanation, but it appears correct to me, as I do not see in the words, *pollon pyreton,* the oppressive heat of the season but rather the many spells of fever that characterize malaria" (p. 64). The hypothesis is, no doubt, acceptable, though it is far from conclusive. The Stoic rhetor Heraclitus proposed a similar explanation (*Homeric Allegories*, VIII, 13) of the plague in Book I of the *Iliad*.

Still to be mentioned is the attribution of human illness to a demonic source, clearly evident in one passage of the *Odyssey*. The shipwrecked Ulysses, riding astride a board, is drifting over the sea at the mercy of the waves. When at the end of three days he sees land it appears to his eyes "as welcome as to his children is the sight of a father's life, who lies in sickness [*nousô*] and strong pains long wasting away, some angry god [*daimôn*] assailing him, if the gods have released him from his trouble [*kakotês*]" (*Od.*, V, 394-98).[12]

From the standpoint of its source illness may be traumatic, divine, environmental, or demonic, and punitive or incomprehensible when its origin is directly divine. But whatever may be its etiology, what *is* illness? What constitutes the distressed state of human reality that we designate by that name? And in the case of the Homeric epic what is, in its author's eyes, the actual nature of the mode of life to which the word *nousos* refers? In a work that can well be considered classic F. E. Clements has classified the various interpretations of illness among so-called primitive peoples.[13] In summary there are three interpretations: illness is conceived of as a loss or escape of the soul of the sufferer, as the magical penetration of an object into his body, or as man's possession by evil spirits. It is not hard to find evidence of the first and the third types in Homer's verses. On the Phaeacian shore the naked Ulysses says that perhaps the cruel frost and the dew of the night "may overcome me, because of my weakness, and I may breathe forth my life [*kekaphêota thymon*]" (*Od.*, V, 463). A possible lethal

12. "Homer applies the term *daimôn*," Nilsson writes, "to anthropomorphic gods of powerful individuality, but more often that individuality is bestowed by the very manifestation of the fate it entails. The fact that the wellspring of man's activity lies within the depths of his soul does not allow him to cite a particular individual god as cause. Man often feels that he is being impelled by an obscure power which opposes his intents and leads him to a final result he has neither prepared nor desired. That power could not be one of individual gods, but is rather some obscure, indeterminate divine power, a *daimôn*" (*Les croyances religieuses de la Grèce antique*, Paris, 1955, p. 72). See also P. Chantraine, "Le divin et les dieux chez Homère," in *La notion du divin depuis Homère jusqu'à Platon* (Vandoeuvres-Genève, 1954).

13. *Primitive Concepts of Disease* (University of California, 1932).

illness from cold is interpreted as a breathing forth or loss of the *thymos;* even though this term, as J. Böhme [14] and B. Snell [15] have shown, may not be equivalent in the epic to *psychê*, it is evident that in the former Homeric expression there lies hidden that primitive vision of the human disease-process as an escape of the soul.[16] And the same idea is no less perceptible in the precise description of the fainting of Sarpedon when he falls wounded (*Il.*, V, 696–98), and of Andromache in the presence of Hector's corpse: both tales attribute the immediate cause of the morbid state to an escape of the *psychê*.

The idea of illness as demonic possession is plainly expressed in the passage from the *Odyssey* quoted above: here the penetration of a hostile *daimôn* consumes the body of the victim in a morbid and painful manner. Can the same be said of the second of the interpretations mentioned: illness as the magical penetration of an object into the body of the sufferer?

Apparently there is nothing in the Homeric epic to recall that crude and primitive view of the disease state. It seems inadmissible to us for Homer's mind to work on such elementary psychological levels, so far from the heights of which Renan was thinking when he spoke of the "Greek miracle." But let us examine attentively the famous description of the plague in Book I of the *Iliad*. Apollo descends from Olympus and from afar, true to his usual epithet, begins to shoot his arrows at the Achaeans: "First did he assail the mules and fleet dogs, but afterward, aiming at the men his piercing darts, he smote" (I,

14. *Die Seele und das Ich im Homerischen Epos* (Leipzig and Berlin, 1929).
15. *Die Entdeckung des Geistes* (Hamburg, 1955). The philosophical and psychological problems posed by the use of the word *psychê* in the Homeric epic are discussed at length in the book by Frenkian mentioned later. See also the chapter, "Origin of the doctrine of the divinity of the soul," in W. Jaeger's book, *La teología de los primeros filósofos griegos* (Spanish translation, México, 1952).
16. *Psychê* is the soul, insofar as the reality thus named keeps man alive, "animates" him; *thymos*, on the other hand, is what causes his movements. See the previously mentioned book by Snell (in the chapter, "Die Auffassung des Menschen bei Homer") for his reasoning in this regard. It need not be explained here in detail.

50–52). Thus a deadly pestilence (*loimos*) ravages the camp of Troy's besiegers, until Achilles has the cause of the plague investigated. Let us now turn aside from the whole matter of Achilles' proposal and the "therapeutic" measures that issue from it; let us concentrate upon the pathogenesis of that devastating plague. Within the concrete and visible reality of the individuals that suffer from it, of what does it consist? What are those arrows that Apollo shoots? Are they the rays of the sun, as the Stoic Heraclitus and other scholiasts of Antiquity suppose, or do they represent bile, as Metrodorus of Lampsacus concluded? [17] It is preferable to abandon allegorical explanations and hold to the immediate sense of the Homeric text. The arrows of Apollo represent the arrival of the causative agent of the disease at the victim's body: a physical though invisible object, the presence of which in the individual receiving it is revealed in the form of material defilement or contamination (*lyma*); a defilement subject to purging lustration by the water of the sea (I, 314). The disease visited by Apollo upon the Achaeans thus consists of a defiling object, a material reality "divinely" superinduced upon the body of the sufferer, in short a physical "stain." [18] The relationship between this conception of the disease state and the idea of the magical intrusion of a foreign and harmful object cannot be denied.[19] Without slighting the brilliant genius of Homer, he

17. The identification of Apollo with the sun was one of the accepted notions of Antiquity; the interpretation of the rhetor Heraclitus is based on it. Metrodorus on the other hand, according to a passage in Philodemus, declared that "Demeter is the liver, Dionysus the spleen and Apollo the bile." See the previously mentioned book by F. Buffière, pp. 127–32 and 195–200.
18. In the case of the plague in the *Iliad* the disease is indeed a "stain." In my book previously cited I have emphasized the ambivalent moral and physical character of this pestilential and punitive stain, as well as the predominance of the importance of the physical aspect of this ambivalence in the interpretation by the Indo-European peoples, and the preponderance of the "moral" aspect in the medical ideology of the Semitic peoples.
19. This relationship between the Homeric conception of the plague and the medical thought of primitive peoples has been spectacularly demonstrated in the following account by Vedder of the *Bergdama* of

was a man of his people and of his time, not an enlightened predecessor of modern science.[20]

II. The Homeric attitude toward the treatment of disease is, as is logical, closely related to this multiform conception of the disease process. But before studying the therapeutic aspect of medicine in the epic, it might perhaps be opportune to consider the view of nature underlying this "nosology"—if the use of a term so unarchaic and coined so long after the way of thinking to which the *Iliad* and the *Odyssey* attest may be permitted—and this "therapy." Medical thought and the idea of Nature are always very directly and immediately interrelated, and Homer's work is no exception to the general rule.

What was Nature to the mind of the Homeric Greek? An inquiry limited merely to the Hellenic name for natural reality, *physis,* cannot give us a definitive answer. The word *physis* is in fact used only once in the epic (*Od.,* X, 303), and with an eloquent yet restricted meaning. More frequently the verb from which this noun is derived appears in Homer's verses— *phyein,* "to grow," "to germinate," "to be born" [21]—as does the adjective *physizoos,* in the sense of "fertile" or "fecund": the earth, in the most noteworthy case (*Il.,* III, 243 and *Od.,* XI, 301). For Homer nature, *Physis,* is thus the whole of all that

---

Southwestern Africa: "*Gamab* is thought of as the god that makes men die and carries them off to their dwelling-place beyond the grave. For this he requires a bow and arrow. A man feeling within himself a serious internal ailment says hopelessly: '*Gamab* has shot me' " (*Die Bergdama,* 1923, p. 103). But this notable similarity between Apollo's and Gamab's methods shows not only the existence of a kinship between the Homeric mentality and that of the *Bergdama;* it reveals also the enormous distance that there is between both peoples. The ancient Greeks' belief is expressed in a splendid work of art, vigorously open to the future: Book I of the *Iliad;* the *Bergdamas'* belief, so coarsely and primitively expressed, remained unchanged as a fossil in the oral tradition of that Negro people until collected and published by an ethnologist.

20. This does not exclude Homer, the father of Greek culture, as the source of Western science. Zubiri would say that Homer made Western science possible but did not foreshadow it, as many of his interpreters naïvely and enthusiastically have thought.

21. The verb *phyô* can be read in *Il.,* IV, 484; VI, 149; XIV, 288; XXI, 352; *Od.,* V, 238, 241, and 477; VII, 114 and 128; IX, 109 and 141; X, 393, etc.

is born and grows, the reality of whatever germinates and takes shape by dint of a creative impulse.

Now things that are born and grow, to whose activity the verb *phyein* can and should be applied, exist in accordance with one of two possible fates: immortality, in the form of permanent and ever-fruitful life, or decrepitude and death. This makes it possible to define within the entire area of reality as Homer sees and comprehends it two distinct though constant and closely interrelated zones: the world of the gods who are born and do not die, and that of beings subsequently to be called "sublunar" who are subject to the sway of corruption and death: clouds and rocks, the waters of the sea, plants, animals, man. For the moment, let us leave the gods in the pure regions of Olympus, and let us try to understand how Homer conceives of the changing reality of things that are born and die.

I do not now propose—let this be clear—to study the genetic relation that may exist between the Homeric view of the reality of the cosmos and the themes of the future *physiologia* of the pre-Socratic thinkers from Thales of Miletus to Anaxagoras and Democritus: whether Homer's *Okeanos*, "the source of everything," did or did not inspire the doctrine of Thales, for whom water is the *arché* or "principle" of *Physis*, whether the Zeus of the *Iliad* is or is not the "air" of Anaximenes and Diogenes of Apollonia, and other such questions.[22] Nor is it my intention to make a descriptive presentation of the idea of the universe implicit in the *Iliad* and the *Odyssey*.[23] In a more

22. The ideas of the ancient Greeks on this genetic relation can be seen in the previously mentioned book by Buffière, that proposed by philologists today in the previously cited work of Onians and in A. M. Frenkian's *Le monde homérique. Essai de protophilosophie grecque* (Paris, 1934).

23. A clear and concise account of the Homeric view of the cosmos may be found in E. Mireaux's *La vie quotidienne au temps d'Homère* (Paris, 1954). Especially fine and thought provoking on this subject is W. Kranz's paper, "Kosmos und Mensch in der Vorstellung frühen Griechentums," in *Nachrichten von der Gesellschaft der Wissenschaften zu Göttingen*, Phil.–hist. Kl., Neue Folge, I, Bd. 2, 1938, p. 121 ff. The book by Frenkian cited in the previous note also contains abundant information on the subject.

modest and immediate fashion I am endeavoring to gather and set in order the features that appear best to define the vision of Nature in the Homeric poems.

The sea and clouds, rivers and plants, animals and men, are frequently described in the pages of the epic. Now in view of all these descriptions, is it possible to identify the particular quality possessed in common by the varied types of reality to which they refer? I believe it is. Such a generic particularity in my opinion is made up of the four following features:

1. *Mutability.* Natural realities are of themselves mutable. To observe them and to describe them in this way is accordingly a very obvious matter: the wind, the sea, and animals *move* in any narrative, ancient and modern, that deals with them. But in addition to the movements that we perceive every day in natural beings, the author of the epic frequently adds others that present-day man would call "out of the ordinary" or "preternatural" if he were willing to be satisfied with noncommittal names: the Xanthus, a river, leaves its bed and pursues Achilles until Hephaestus sends forth a great flame against it (*Il.*, XXI, 331–84); Achilles' horse, also named Xanthus, speaks to the hero and prophesies his death (*Il.*, XIX, 400–20); Circe turns men into swine with magic drugs (*Od.*, X, 229–43); Poseidon with his trident cleaves the rock on which Ajax had seated himself (*Od.*, IV, 499–509); and much else of the same.

2. *The "divinity" of the properties and movements of natural beings.* What I have said previously would seem to indicate that the Homeric epic distinguishes two classes of movements in the visible world: those which are natural or spontaneous and those produced by the direct action of the gods. This is certainly true, but it is not the whole truth. Bruno Snell has called attention to the "naturalness" of the acts of divine intervention in the *Iliad* and the *Odyssey*, both those concerning the conduct of men—for example, Pallas Athene's role in the dispute between Achilles and Agamemnon (Il., I, 195–218) —as well as those affecting nonhuman realities. Snell gives a good illustration of this character of the Homeric—more gen-

erally of the Hellenic—mind by pointing out the contrast between the attitude of the Greeks and of the Israelites toward augury: "For the Greeks the way that Gideon deals with his God in the Book of Judges (IV, 36–40) would have been surprising. The favor of God is revealed in such a case by a violation of natural law; for God nothing is impossible. In the Greek legends, too, it may be that the heroes ask for visible signs of divine aid, but such signs are a stroke of lightning, a bird's flight, a sneeze—all things that admittedly, according to the laws of probability, may not happen at a desired moment, but which, it might always be said, could well occur because of a fortunate change, *agathê tykhê*. To the way of thinking of a classic Greek, the gods themselves are subject to the order of the universe, and in Homer they always intervene in a natural manner. Even when Hera forces Helios to plunge quickly into the Ocean the event continues to be natural, since Helios, thought of as a charioteer, can on occasion make his horses run faster." [24] This shrewd observation by Snell seems confirmed in the contrary sense by the use of the adjective "divine" (*theios*) to express the outstanding efficacy of some natural realities: salt ("divine salt" it is called in *Il.*, IX, 214) or wine ("drink of the gods," *Od.*, II, 341). The gods act upon the visible world in a natural way and some things of the visible world are "divine"; and "divine" things, also naturally divine, are the most banal and everyday phenomena of Nature such as the dawn (*Êôs*) or the wind (*Aiolos*). The conclusion is inescapable: in the Homeric world there is no gap between those movements of the cosmos that seem spontaneous and those that the will of the gods directly causes, or, more concisely, between the natural and the divine. The phrase, "everything is full of gods," attributed to Thales by Aristotle (*de anima*, I, 5, 411a 7), doubtlessly has a much more ancient origin than in the work of the philosopher of Miletus.

3. *Perishability.* The beings of the visible world are perishable. In a rock as in a man, natural movement ends in death and extinction. At the core of the strong light of the Hellenic

---

24. "Der Glaube an die olympischen Götter," p. 49.

world unconquerable melancholy lies hidden. It is impossible not to recall here the famous words of Glaucus to Diomedes: "Even as are the generations of leaves, such are those likewise of men; the leaves that be, the wind scattereth on the earth, and the forest buddeth and putteth forth more again, when the season of spring is at hand; so of the generations of men, one putteth forth and another ceaseth" (*Il.*, VI, 146–49).

4. *Incipient "regularity."* The movement of natural realities, though divine, is not capricious: it has an inner regularity at once deep-seated and obvious when it is observed calmly and accurately. Certainly the accuracy with which the eyes of Homer—blind in his old age, according to tradition—were able to view the visible world was not inconsiderable. It suffices to collect the epithets in the epic that express the appearance of the sea, as did Finsler, or to read the detailed description of the wounds suffered by Phereklos (*Il.*, V, 59–68) and Aeneas (*Il.*, V, 297–311), or follow the tale of the fall of Antinoos, mortally wounded by Ulysses' arrow, to note with astonishment the sharpness and accuracy of the poet's vision, never equaled in any of the other epic narratives of humanity. Not in vain does he tell us, in praise of the Achaeans, that they are *helikôpes*, men of sharp and lively eyes (*Il.*, I, 389). One who can observe perceptible reality with such minuteness must necessarily note in it the existence of deep-seated regularities, not only in the course of the stars and the rhythm of vegetation but also in man's influence upon natural processes accessible to him and in the operative powers of beings that are born and die on earth. Surgical technique in the *Iliad* is implicitly governed by the following principle: "If in the living reality of the wounded human body such-and-such a thing is done, it will have such-and-such a result"; this is nothing else than a description of Nature's regularity in regard to the reactions of the human body. But where this discovery of the essential relationship between appearance and specific quality—the prime basis of the future "scientific" vision of Nature—is most clearly and decisively revealed is in the verses where Homer describes the herb that is to free Ulysses from Circe's spell:

"When he had spoken thus," says Ulysess, "Hermes gave me the plant that he had plucked from the ground, and he showed me the nature [*physis*] thereof. It was black at the root, but the flower was like to milk. *Môly* the gods call it, and it is very hard for mortal men to dig" (*Od.*, X, 302–06). It is not necessary to emphasize the significance and importance of this passage, the only one in the epic in which the word *physis* appears. With this word, the poet designates a reality characterized by three features: it is born and grows and hence can be named with a word derived from the verb *phyein*; it has a constant shape, subject to precise description; it contains an operative power, that of preventing the effect of Circe's magic drugs. In short, the regularity with which a visible outward appearance reveals the latent existence of a particular quality is called *physis*.[25] The *physiologia* of the Ionic thinkers and, moreover, of Greek philosophy and Western natural science takes its primary origin from these simple words of Homer. Let us not view Homer as the first man of science of the West, as others have naïvely viewed him, as the first hygienist or the first military surgeon; let us rather view him as the man through whom the way of thought that made European science possible first finds expression. Our praise is not thereby lessened and is much more to the point.

III. Perceptible reality reveals itself to the eyes of Homer as changeable, divinely moved, perishable, and regular. This, then, is the framework and basis of what we might call the "therapeutic idea" of the epic. To introduce this subject, let us first look at the various practices in which it is revealed.

Most of these belong to the three categories of the art of healing that later Greek thought was to distinguish: surgical, pharmaceutical or medicinal, and dietetic.[26] I need not again

25. The term *eidos* in the sense of the form or *appearance* of a thing appears several times in the Homeric epic (*Il.*, II, 58 and III, 39; *Od.*, XVII, 454, etc.). *Il.*, II, 58 connects the appearance (*eidos*), the bulk, and the lusty stature (*phyê*) of a human figure, very similar to Nestor, seen in dreams. *Eidos* and *megethos* indicate the *physis*, the character or "nature" of that which is born and grows.

26. The antiquity of this triple division of medical art—see gloss from Venetus B on *Il.*, XI, 515; Plato, *Rep.* III, 405d–07d—has been oppor-

reproduce and discuss the Homeric passages in which there is allusion to surgical practices, curative drugs, or dietetic prescriptions, the less so since a consideration of all these measures against disease is in a way outside my present scope, the study of the therapeutic word. I shall limit myself to referring the reader to the publications previously cited. On the other hand, I must carefully inquire into two other therapeutic practices much less studied by writers: catharsis and spells.

Description of cathartic practices, or at least allusion to them, is frequent in the *Iliad* and the *Odyssey* (see Moulinier's monograph mentioned previously). But is there among these practices any one the purpose of which is to purify and hence cure a man of the disease from which he suffers? This is the urgent problem posed by the conduct of the Achaeans in the face of the plague in Book I of the *Iliad*. Let us review it. Moved by the gravity of the epidemic, Achilles calls the Danaans together and speaks thus: "Let us inquire of some soothsayer or priest, yea, or an interpreter of dreams—seeing that dreams, too, are of Zeus—who shall say wherefore Phoebus Apollo is so wroth, whether he blame us by reason of vow or hecatomb; if perchance he would accept the savour of lambs or unblemished goats, and so would take away the pestilence from us." To this, the augur Kalchas, son of Thestor, replies: "He who smiteth afar . . . will never remove the loathly pestilence from the Danaans till we have given the bright-eyed damsel to her father and carried a holy hecatomb to Chryses." Achilles and Agamemnon dispute about the matter, Pallas Athene and Nestor intervene, Atreides finally gives in, and Ulysses leaves for Chrysê, taking with him the damsel and the victims for propitiatory sacrifice. But Atreides also "ordered the men to purify themselves [*apolymainesthai*], and they purified themselves and cast the defilements into the sea and did sacrifice to Apollo, even unblemished hecatombs of bulls and goats,

---

tunely emphasized by W. Artelt in *Studien zur Geschichte der Medizin*, Leipzig, 1937, pp. 41–42. Plato's contrary opinion in the passage cited does not rule out the use of dietetic means for curative purposes in the epic: see what is later said regarding Machaon's cure by Nestor.

along the shore of the solitary sea." Chryses in turn receives Ulysses' mission and asks Apollo to put an end to his wrath: "Remove thou from the Danaans forthwith the loathly pestilence," he says at the end of his prayer. The hecatomb and the hymns that Ulysses and his men offer the god also play a part in the process: "All day long the Achaeans appeased the god with music, singing a beautiful paean to Apollo, the Far-Darter; and his heart was glad to hear." And so the plague that had been ravaging the Danaan camp ends.

In the face of the plague decimating them, the Achaeans adopt a therapeutic behavior—let us choose this term in preference to "treatment," much more modern in attitude—in which may be distinguished three features: the prompt termination of the state of injustice that had brought on the disease as punishment, the propitiation of the angry god, in this case Apollo, and the purifying lustration. Agamemnon returns Chryseis to her father, Apollo receives a tribute of hecatombs and prayers, and the Achaean hosts purify themselves by bathing in the sea.

Let us now restrict ourselves to the examination of this last practice. Is the bath prescribed by Atreides for his men a true religious and moral *katharsis,* a rite of purification? Körner roundly denies this: "The purification of the people and the casting of the impurity into the sea," he writes, "was merely a hygienic measure, for if it had been an act aimed at propitiation of the god it would be impossible to understand why the people affected by the plague were purified, rather than the guilty prince who by his behavior brought on the epidemic." [27] A similar objection, even though not based on the question of the lustral bath, was current among ancient commentators. Zoilus in particular emphasized the inconsistency of Apollo, who should have punished Agamemnon rather than the anonymous mass of soldiers many of whom surely had desired the restitution of Chryseis. Moreover, the god causes widespread death even among beasts of burden and dogs, poor creatures that had nothing to do with the abduction of the daughter of

27. O. Körner, *Wesen und Wert der homerischen Heilkunde* (Wiesbaden, 1904), p. 12.

Chryses.[28] Stengel is even more radical: according to him, Homer probably was never acquainted with a *katharsis* of magic character.[29] Conditioned by their "enlightened" veneration for the Homeric poems, neither Körner nor Stengel can admit that their author would pay homage to so archaic and irrational a way of thought as is attested to by rites of purification. Rather than a ritual purification, they deem the Achaeans' bath a mere cleansing.

Among philologists and religious historians, however—Wächter, Nilsson, Dodds—the attribution of a strictly cathartic character to the bath of Troy's besiegers has prevailed.[30] Dodds, for example, says: "It seems quite clear that the purifications described in *Il.*, I, 314, and in *Od.*, XXII, 481, are cathartic in nature, in the magical sense of the word, in one case for the elimination of *lymata* (impurities), and in the other because of the description of sulfur as *kakôn akos* (cure of evils)." Zoilus' and Körner's moral objection cannot be taken into account. Apollo punishes Agamemnon not with the plague, but with the threat of catastrophic defeat of his undertaking; he punishes him further in the persons of those who are in close tribal relation to him. As Glotz showed, the freeing of the individual from family and tribal bonds is a relatively late event in the history of Greek culture.[31] To an archaic mind, the sin of Agamemnon was a sin of Agamemnon's people, and in one way or another divine punishment must fall upon that entire people.[32]

28. Heraclitus, *Homeric Allegories,* XIV, 22. A gloss of Venetus A on *Il.* I, 50, seeks to solve the problem by saying that the god begins by smiting the animals as a warning: he does not wish to exterminate the Greeks but merely to give them a lesson.
29. P. Stengel: "Opferblut und Opfergerste," *Hermes, 41* (1906), 230–46.
30. Th. Wächter, "Reinheitsvorschriften im griechischen Kult," *Religionsgeschichtliche Vorarbeiten und Versuche,* 9, 1910; M. P. Nilsson, *Geschichte der griechischen Religion,* p. 82, and *Griechische Feste von religiöser Bedeutung* (Leipzig, 1906), p. 99; E. R. Dodds, pp. 35 and 54.
31. G. Glotz, *La solidarité de la famille dans le droit criminel en Grèce* (Paris, 1904).
32. Plato still speaks of "the diseases and most horrible trials which, as a result of ancient offenses, and without their origin being known, afflict some lineages" (*Phaedrus* 244d). Exactly the same opinion is to

But writers are apt to ignore the clearly "therapeutic" character of that lustral bath. Moulinier, for example, writes: "As soon as Agamemnon has bidden the restitution of Chryseis to her father he orders his troops to cleanse themselves [*apolymainesthai*]. This act is a prelude to the hecatomb about to be offered to Apollo. Before praying it is necessary to wash." [33] This observation is unobjectionable: as in so many other passages of the epic, lustration or *katharsis* must precede prayer and sacrifice; in order to deal with the gods, one must be pure, and cleanliness is nothing else than the outer sign of purity. But in our case this is not the whole truth, because it has been forgotten that when Agamemnon orders the lustral bath the plague in the Achaean camp has not yet ceased. Kalchas has declared that Apollo "will not remove the loathly pestilence from the Danaans till we have given the bright-eyed damsel to her father, unbought, unransomed, and carried a holy hecatomb to Chryse; once we have appeased him thus our hope will be reborn" (*Il.*, I, 97–100). Now in fact it happens that the Achaeans' lustration precedes both the actual return of Chryseis and the twofold hecatomb with which the god is propitiated: one that will be offered jointly by Agamemnon and the soldiery of his armies and one that will be sacrificed by the twenty men under the command of Ulysses who are to carry the maiden to Chryse. Moreover, these men, as yet untouched by the plague and among whom Atreides had to choose (*Il.*, I, 309), purify themselves by means of prayer and the ritual sprinkling of barley meal before their hecatomb (*Il.*, I, 458) rather than by lustration in the water of the sea. The lustral ceremony seems to be reserved to those who are

be found in *Il.*, IV, 160 ff; Hesiod, *Works and Days*, p. 333; Solon, frag. 1 Diehl 30–32, etc. When the awareness of individual personality awakens, its collision with this belief will give rise to a common tragic situation: a man who feels innocent finds himself punished: see the next chapter.

33. P. 26. Nilsson is of the same opinion: "After the plague, the Achaeans purify the camp and cast the *lymata* [impurities] into the sea before making sacrifice." In *Geschichte der griechischen Religion;* the passage quoted can be found on pp. 85–86 of the English translation by Fielden (2d ed, Oxford, 1949).

impure because of the *lymata* of the disease. In other words: the Achaeans' bath in Book I of the *Iliad* is cathartic in a twofold sense: it ritually prepares for the sacrifice the men who are about to offer it, and it does so by cleansing or purifying them of the impurity or physical defilement (*lyma*) through which the punishment inflicted by Apollo attains perceptible and disease-causing reality. The treatment of the plague is cathartic in nature, and catharsis in such cases has an aim simultaneously ritual and therapeutic. Those stricken with the plague in the *Iliad* "treat"—if such a term may be allowed—their ailment by washing their bodies and appeasing the gods with prayer and sacrifice.[34]

The therapeutic use of charms or conjurations (*epôdê*) also has an indubitably magic character. Only once is it mentioned in the Homeric epic. Ulysses, while hunting with the sons of Autolycus, is wounded in the leg by a wild boar. His hunting companions gather around him, skillfully bind up (*dêsan*) his wound and by means of a charm (*epaoidê*) stanch the flow of dark blood (*Od.*, XIX, 457). In this treatment one purely medical aspect, the skillful bandaging of the wound, and another genuinely magical, the reciting of the charm, are usually distinguished. But Scheftelowitz and Pfister have called attention to the fact that both the Greek verb *deô*, "bind" or "tie," as well as the Latin *ligare*, frequently designate the act of enchanting by tying or binding.[35] "Diseases and wounds, even though their cause may be obvious," writes Pfister, "are usually attributed to the action of malign demons; this was the general belief. By means of bindings they can be fettered and their action hindered; this in my opinion is the sense of *dêsan*. To the effect of the binding that of a charm or *epôdê* is

---
34. Elsewhere (*Introducción histórica al estudio de la patología psicosomática*) I have emphasized the significance of the primarily physical character of the therapeutic purification described by the author of the *Iliad*.

35. Scheftelowitz, "Das Schlingen und Netzmotiv im Glauben und Brauch der Völker," *Religionsgeschichtliche Vorarbeiten und Versuche*, 12, 2; H. Pfister, "Epode," in the *Realencyclopädie* of Pauly-Wissowa, Suppl. Bd. 4, 325.

joined." Thus the intervention of the sons of Autolycus must have had a purely and exclusively magic character from start to finish and is plainly one more proof of the demonic conception of disease.[36]

The Greek word for "charm" or "conjuration" (*epaoidê, epôdê*) enters history with the above-mentioned verse of the *Odyssey*, but the use of charms or conjurations with therapeutic intent—verbal formulas of magic character, recited or chanted in the presence of the patient to achieve his cure—has belonged, perhaps ever since the Paleolithic age, to almost all forms of so-called primitive culture.[37] It therefore appears necessary to suppose that the *epaoidê* of the sons of Autolycus is literary evidence for a much more ancient tradition, as deeply rooted in Mycenaean and Cretan culture as in the customs of the Doric invaders. From those remote sources of Greek culture to the final years of its Hellenistic period, the magic *epôdê* was never to lose its force in the popular medicine of Hellas and was always to have a character oscillating between that of a conjuration and that of a charm. It becomes a conjuration with predominance of an intent to command or coerce the realities to be modified or avoided (such as a flow of blood or the action of a devil), a charm when its intent is predominantly entreaty or supplication. In the latter case its efficacy seems to depend not only upon the formula of the charm itself and the "power" or "virtue" of the person, whether priest or common man, employing it, but also in the final instance upon the divine powers that hear the speaker's words.

We cannot know what the contents of the *epaoidê* of the sons of Autolycus may have been; but if what the Hellenic *epaoidê* was in later centuries be borne in mind it does not

36. Recall the passage, also from the *Odyssey* (V, 394–98), which I have cited above.
37. See *A History of Medicine*, by H. E. Sigerist, vol. 1 (New York, 1951), 191–216; the articles "Zauber" and "Zauberarzt" (Thurnwald, Roeder, Sudhoff) in the *Reallexikon der Vorgeschichte*, ed. by Max Ebert (Berlin, 1929); and *La medicina primitiva*, by A. Pazzini (Rome, 1941). On the conjurations of shamanism, including European shamanism, see M. Eliade, *Le chamanisme et les techniques archaïques de l'extase* (Paris, 1951).

seem venturesome to suppose that language and music played a role. A verbal formula chanted or sung: that is what the charm with which Ulysses' wound was "treated" must have been. Whether or not its mention in the *Odyssey* is related to the *epôdai* of the Orphic tradition is a matter that perhaps may never be decided. Only this is certain: that charms for therapeutic purpose already existed at the birth of Greek culture. The next chapter will show their presence and final form in the post-Homeric period of this culture.

But in Homer's epic the therapeutic word is not always a magic epôdê. A careful reading of the *Iliad* and the *Odyssey* discloses in their pages two other ways of using verbal expression to effect the cure of a patient or aid toward it: the non-magical plea for health, in the form of a prayer to the gods, and a persuasive and strengthening conversation with the patient.

The paean Ulysses and his fellow sailors raise to Apollo to allay the god's wrath against the Achaeans (*Il.*, X, 473) is a clear and excellent example of the supplicatory use of language in order to cure disease; no less evident is this mental attitude in the Cyclops' allusion to a possible prayer by Polyphemus to Poseidon, if his ailment is not caused by a visible act of violence (*Od.*, IX, 412). In contrast to the *epaoidê*, with its more or less coercive intention, the *euchê* of the Achaeans and Cyclops is limited to pure supplication. The speaker of the charm always endeavors to compel Nature in some measure. I have previously remarked that there is an unbroken transition between charm and conjuration; one who prays, on the contrary, merely *asks* the gods for a favorable course of natural events.[38]

[38]. This, however, does not oppose the existence of an unbroken transition between the *epôdê* and the *euchê* in the works of classical antiquity. Sometimes the same imprecation is called *epôdê* by some authors and *euchê* by others. Thus (Pfister, p. 325) the words spoken by Croesus on the pyre to put out the fire are called *epôdê* by Herodotus (I, 87) and Xanthus (FHG, I, 41s), and *euchê* by Eustatius. It also occurs that followers of one religious belief call the incantations or charms of other faiths *epôdai*, and their own, *euchai*. This was to be the practice of both pagans and Christians in their debates with one another.

In sharp contrast to charm and prayer with respect to their curative intention are the words addressed by Nestor to Machaon and by Patroclus to Eurypylus, when both find it necessary to treat the wounds inflicted upon their comrades. Nestor bears Machaon to his tent, fortifies him with a mixture of Pramnian wine, grated goatsmilk cheese, and barley flour prepared by the slave Hekamêdê, and the two men divert one another with their tales, *mythoisin terponto* (*Il.*, XI, 643). Patroclus, on his part, expertly treats Eurypylus' arrow wound and entertains him with words during his skilled surgical operation: "Patroclus sat in the tent of brave Eurypylus, and was making him glad with talk, and on his cruel wound was laying herbs, to medicine his dark pain" (*Il.*, XV, 392-94).

Human speech is therapeutically used in both cures for a purpose completely different from the two previous instances: it is no longer a charm or supplication but rather the deliberate utilization of some of the psychological or, better, psychosomatic effects that human speech can produce upon the hearer, in this case amusing or cheering the mind (*terpô*). Nestor and Patroclus—the latter more obviously, according to the text of the poem—speak to their patients so that the diverting effect of the words they then utter may contribute in some way to the proper execution and the success of their therapeutic procedure. It might also be said of this instance that the therapist's words aid in the treatment by "charming" the patient, but that charm is not a product of the magic power a given verbal formula may possess, such as is typical of a charmer's chant. Rather it is, in the usual figurative sense of the word, the persuasive delight that an utterance delightful

---

The subject will be taken up again at a later point in this book. For the moment let it suffice to note the gradual transition between the *epôdê*-conjuration, in which the aim at a coercive effect is greatest, and the *euchê* or prayer, in which there is merely supplication, with the *epôdê*-charm as the middle stage.

The term *euchê* is used in the Homeric epic once only, when Circe bids Ulysses offer prayers to the dead (*Od.*, X, 526); but in other forms (the nouns *euchos* and *euchôlê*, the verb *euchomai*) this same root is relatively frequent in the *Iliad* and the *Odyssey*. I think, therefore, that the foregoing remarks are entirely legitimate.

"of itself" produces as a result of its very meaning in the soul of one listening to it. In contrast to the presumption of the "magical" effect of the spoken word, so evident in the *epaoidê* of the sons of Autolycus, in the epic a conscious "natural" use of the psychological effect human speech possesses of itself is suggested.[39]

IV. The spoken word is used in the Homeric epic with respect to disease for three different purposes: for supplication, for magical effect, and with a psychological or natural aim. The language of supplication is the "prayer" (*euchê*), of magic the "charm" (*epôdê*), for a psychological purpose "pleasant speech" (*terpnos logos*) or "beguiling" speech (*thelktêrios logos*). Let us study in greater detail the particular nature and structure of the two last ways of curing by speaking.

As I have already remarked, the practice called by the Greeks *epôdê*, "conjuration" or "charm," is present in almost all primitive or archaic cultures as soon as they attain the relative degree of complexity that "magical" precision requires *vis-à-vis* the reality of the world. Societies leading a rudimentary existence, hunting and food-gathering peoples for example, do not practice magic and seem to give very little attention to illness: a sick person is usually abandoned to his fate, often in the most literal way by being left alone somewhere in the forest.[40] The situation is quite different once agriculture

---

39. The Spanish verb *encantar*—as well as corresponding terms in other languages: *enchanter, incantare,* etc.—is derived from the *incantamenta* or "incantations" of the Romans, and is semantically and morphologically parallel to the Greek verb *epadein:* as in the former the prefix *in,* so in the latter the prefix *epi* refers to the "chant" (*cantum, ôdê*) of which the charm or conjuration consisted. To say *epôdê* in Greek is the same as saying *incantamentum* in Latin. From that original meaning comes the weaker, nonmagical sense of the Spanish *encantar,* the French *enchanter,* and the Italian *incantare*—meanings quite similar to those possessed as a result of a like process by *bewitch* in English and *bezaubern* or *behexen* in German.

40. See the works previously indicated, particularly the book by H. E. Sigerist, and the article by Thurnwalt in Ebert's *Reallexikon*. This is not to say that in the most primitive societies attitudes toward disease more or less close to that expressed in the Greek *epôdê* do not occur.

and animal husbandry have won social importance, and even more so with the dawn of those ways of living that we today call "historical cultures"—those of Egypt, Sumer, or the pre-Hellenic civilizations. The therapeutic charm then visibly thrives in a wide variety of forms and with the most diverse contents. Quite different, for example, are the charms Gutmann has collected among the African *dschagga*, those observed by Preuss among the American Indians, and those that Assyriologists, Egyptologists, and Hellenists have been publishing for some time.[41] But despite their diversity, apparent in all of them is an attempt to compel Nature, by reciting or chanting a particular verbal formula, to perform what is desired of her: the curing of a disease, rainfall, or the success of a hunting expedition.

From this common trunk grow the *epaoidai* of the sons of Autolycus and the *epôdai* so often mentioned in later Greek literature. Until the proper time for the study of the latter comes, here are the principal characteristic traits with which therapeutic enchantment appears in the Hellenic world:

1. In contrast with what occurs in other cultures, the recitation of a therapeutic charm does not appear to be the exclusive privilege of the members of a particular caste of priests, shamans, or medicine men. It is likely that the recitation of charms was not foreign to the magic and religious practice of the *arêtêres*, or priests, mentioned in the *Iliad* as imploring the gods (I, 11, and V, 78), but there is no indication that Autolycus and his sons had any special priestly qualifications. We only know that the former, the maternal grandfather of Ulysses, "excelled other men in stealing and swearing, gifts that Hermes himself had bestowed upon him" (*Od.*, XIX, 396–97);

---

41. Gutmann, *Dichten und Denken der Dschagga-Neger*, 1909; Preuss, *Psychologische Forschungen II*, 1922; Contenau, *La médecine en Assyrie et en Babylonie*, 1938; Wiedemann, *Magie und Zauberei im alten Ägypten*, 1905. The first to note the importance of the *epôdê* in Greek culture was F. G. Welcker, in his article, "Epode oder die Besprechung," *Kleine Schriften III* (Bonn, 1850). Pfister's above-mentioned article in the *Realencyclopädie* of Pauly-Wissowa is the best philological treatment on the subject of the *epôdê*.

as regards the second of these gifts, this may perhaps have some bearing on his possession of a special power to charm diseases and wounds.[42]

2. The words of which the charm consisted were not addressed to the person of the patient. What was directly and immediately chanted in this case—what the magical chant was aimed at—was not the man suffering the ailment, but the powers that ruled over the activities of Nature in a normal way or in an anomalous situation. The sons of Autolycus recite their *epaoidê* to stanch the bleeding of Ulysses' wound and address their charm to the power controlling the hemorrhage, to the *daimôn* intended to be "bound" or "tied" in a magical way by the bandage, if Pfister's interpretation is correct.[43]

3. The supposed mechanism of magical action attributed to the *epaoidê* or *incantamentum* seems very different from the word magic practiced by other peoples, the Semites in particular. The Assyrians and Babylonians, for example, believed that he who knew the "true" names of things and of the devils that change them had magic power: by pronouncing the true name of a thing one becomes its master and can control it. The metaphysical significance of names in Semitic thought constitutes the basis for this idea of the control of reality through magic.[44] But this does not apply to the magical incantation of

[42]. *Horkos*, "oath," literally means, "that which confines and obliges." See Aeschylus (*Agam.*, 1198–99): "And how could an oath, no matter how sincere and firm, cure the ill?" The passage refers to the curse afflicting the descendants of Atreus; and even though denying that the act of swearing has sufficient power to cure this family of its terrible fate, the phrase evidently assumes belief in *some sort of* healing effect of swearing upon various punitive ills, disease among them. On this subject see the following chapter.

[43]. All practice of magic is an attempt to "oblige" Nature. This term is all the more suitable, inasmuch as the word "oblige"—from *ob-ligare* —contains within it a magical source. It comes from the Roman practice of magically "binding" a thing to "oblige" it to do what was sought of it. See the previously mentioned work by Scheftelwitz.

[44]. For the therapeutic conjurations and charms of the Assyrians and Babylonians, consult the previously cited book by Contenau (pp. 146 ff). "'Biblical metaphysics,' writes C. Tresmontant, 'is a metaphysics of the name, of the proper name. "I have known thee by thy name" (*Ex.*, 33, 12, 17, and numerous other verses) . . . Particular beings are loved

the Greeks. The supposed efficacy of the latter does not come from secretly and magically "naming" reality—recall the "Open, Sesame!" of the Arabian tales—but from charming or seducing the mind of the divine invisible powers governing the process to be modified; this is the reason why the verbal formula of the Greek incantations is not customarily a secret language but rather a functional expression more or less in harmony with the nature of the end to be achieved. What is said of the paean sung by Ulysses and his men in Book I of the *Iliad*—"Apollo heard them with contented heart" (I, 474)—could be said again, changing the circumstances, of the *epaoidê* with which the hero's wound is treated in the *Odyssey*.

4. The possible relationship between the therapeutic charm and catharsis: Did the *epaoidê* of the sons of Autolycus have any purifying effect? Nothing seems to indicate this in the passage describing it. We know, however, that words and chants are very frequently purifying devices [45]—we shall soon have occasion to offer proof of this in the later history of Greek culture—and it is not improbable that the author of that passage may have attributed to a *daimôn* a decisive role in the origin of the hemorrhage to be stanched. In such a case the charm, the application of which was aimed at expelling or ending the action of the harmful *daimôn*, must have possessed some purifying power in the minds of those who used it.

Essentially distinct from the magic *epaoidê* is, as we have seen, the therapeutic use of the human word previously designated "persuasive" or "cheering." Aware of the great prestige possessed by speech and its various psychological processes in

---

and created for their own sake. Their proper name, in essence, is unique and irreplaceable. Each being is, as Laberthonnière puts it, a *hapax legomenon*. This metaphysics of the proper name is obviously directly antithetical to individuation by matter and lies at the source of Christian personalism' (*La pensée hebraïque*, Paris, 1953, p. 100). For the Semite, the 'word' (*dabar*) is creation: God created the world by uttering the 'name' of things, and a man who knows their 'true names' does the same thing, within his limitations and in his own way."

45. Pfister, "Katharsis," in Pauly-Wissowa, Suppl. Bd. 4, 159.

the epic, can anyone be surprised that the Homeric heroes are familiar with and use the persuasive power of the human word upon the mind of a listener? Achilles, by his father's design, is educated both in fair speech and in outstanding valor (*Il.*, X, 443); Eumaeus places the bard among those who perform useful duties for the people (*Od.*, XVII, 385); Phemius, likened to the gods themselves because of his talent for song (*Od.*, I, 371), owes his life to that ability (*Od.*, XXII, 330); the tales of Demodocus, the Phaeacian bard, delight men and make them weep (*Od.*, VIII, passim); Ulysses proclaims the honor and veneration that men everywhere render to bards (*Od.*, VIII, 479-80). The whole epic is in a way an enthusiastic homage to superiority in the use of words and their power to touch men's hearts.[46] I repeat my previous question: can it be surprising that Nestor and Patroclus utilize the efficacy of cheering speech to quiet the souls of their patients?

Let us note the initial peculiarity of this new type of therapeutic word. There seem to be two chief features that characterize it:

1. In contrast to what occurs with prayers and incantations, cheering speech is addressed to the patient as a human individual; not to his innermost moral being, however, as in the rit-

---

46. The act of enchanting or seducing (*thelgô*) by means of speech, and hence the conception of the word as a means of magical seduction (*thelktêrion*), are frequent in the Homeric epic, particularly in the *Odyssey*. Aphrodite's belt contains the enchantment or witchery of sweet dialogues of love (*Od.*, XIV, 215); Calypso detains Ulysses by bewitching him with tender and seductive words (*Od.*, I, 57); Phêmius enchants men with his accounts of deeds of prowess by men and gods (*Od.*, I, 337); Aegisthus was able to enchant or seduce Agamemnon's wife with his words (*Od.*, III, 264); the sirens bewitch men with their singing (*Od.*, XII, 40); a man of Aetolia deceives Eumaeus with the seduction of his words (*Od.*, XIV, 387); Eumaeus tells Penelope of a guest—Ulysses—whose tales will enchant her heart (*Od.*, XVII, 514); the bard's recitation enchants mortal men (*Od.*, XVII, 521); with her sweet words Penelope has cunningly succeeded in seducing her suitors' minds (*Od.*, XVIII, 282). From its very beginnings, Greek culture is a culture of the *logos*, speech, now in a magical, now in a rational sense. Nevertheless Greek medicine was incapable of developing verbal psychotherapy of a "technical" type. In subsequent chapters this curious inability will become evident.

ual interrogations of Assyrian medicine, but rather to his mind or *thymos*, that is, to the element within him capable of producing affective and somatic activity. The Assyrian *bârû* spoke to the "person" of the patient; Nestor and Patroclus speak to the individual "nature" of their patient. Once again the contrast between the personal orientation of the Semitic mentality and the natural orientation of the Greek mentality becomes evident.[47]

2. The cheering speech of Nestor and Patroclus exercises its particular therapeutic action by means of the natural efficacy possessed by what they say, not because of some presumed magic power in their speech. Thus the curative process of the *terpnos logos* (cheering speech) is natural in a twofold sense: both as a result of its own character and because of the reality upon which it acts. The therapist in this case speaks so that his words, by acting upon the nature of the patient, may produce in it an effect natural to them. Homer designates as the *physis* of the *môly*, the plant that can protect against Circe's enchantments, the regularity with which the configuration of this plant reveals its character and hidden properties. Could not the "natural" quality possessed by the therapeutic action of cheering speech then be rightly defined by stating that its *physis* consists in the regularity with which its acoustic effect upon the senses—the words and their intonation—reveals its latent property of working a favorable change in the minds of those in need who hear it?

Let us now view as a whole the variegated picture of medical thought and methods of treatment displayed in the *Iliad* and the *Odyssey*. Disease may be traumatic, environmental, demonic, and punitive, and in the last case either with or without a preceding transgression on the part of the sufferer. In turn, therapy takes the most varied forms: it is alternately or simultaneously surgical, pharmaceutical, dietetic, cathartic or purifying, and verbal; and in the final case with magic intent or by strictly natural means. The Homeric view of Nature

---

47. Again, I refer the reader to the book by Contenau mentioned above, and to my *Introducción al estudio de la patología psicosomática*.

sketched above provides the background for this picture: a changing, transient reality with movement subject to determinants and influences of widely diverse character, but within which the human mind is beginning to glimpse a basic and immanent regularity. Thales of Miletus and Anaximander are indeed quite far removed from men who see Eos, the spouse of Tithonus, behind the dawn, and the wrath of Poseidon behind angry waves of the tempest; but on the other hand Thales of Miletus and Anaximander are possible and even probable in the future of a society that designates as *physis* the set of visible features by which the nature of a plant is revealed, just as Socrates and Plato are possible and probable in the spiritual lineage of men who have begun to value and understand in such a lofty way the excellence of the human word. The Greek culture of the centuries subsequent to the composition of the Homeric epic will show us how the possibilities contained in the rich inexhaustible web of its verses are fulfilled, or remain unfulfilled, in the therapeutic use of the word.

Chapter 2

From Homer to Plato

Faced with the distressing fact of disease, Homeric man made purposeful or religious use of drugs, surgery, dietetic remedies, rites of purification, and words. Logotherapy is as ancient as Western culture itself. But, as we have seen, the curative word—by this I mean the use of the spoken word to achieve the cure of a patient—acquired in the Homeric world three forms quite distinct from one another: the "prayer" (*euchê*), the "charm" or "conjuration" (*epôdê*), and "persuasive" or "cheering" speech (*terpnos, thelktêrios logos*). The preceding pages have revealed the existence of an unbroken transition from the prayer to the charm; this, of course, does not deny the reality of pure forms of both in more ancient modes of life. The present chapter in turn will reveal to our eyes the historical process of the gradual approach of the *epôdê*, or at least of one way of interpreting the *epôdai*, to the "persuasive" word. But before this process is taken up in detail, it will be well to consider as a whole the period in which it begins.

I. From the eighth until well into the fifth century B.C.—between Homer and Pericles if names be preferred to dates—a major change affecting all spheres of human existence occurs in Greek life: religiosity, social life, the relationship between man and material things, the attitude of the individual toward his own reality. Using the terminology of the American anthropologists, Dodds speaks of the transition from a culture of "point of honor" to a culture of "guilt"; the "shame culture" of the epic turns into a "guilt culture." [1] "If a good warrior receives no more honor [*timê*] than a poor warrior, why fight?"

1. Dodds, *The Greeks*, pp. 18 and 28–63. For reasons later indicated I have translated "shame culture" as *cultura del pundonor* (culture of

Achilles says on one occasion (*Il.*, IX, 315 ff). "I am ashamed before the men of Troy [*aideomai Trôas*]," cries Hector before departing for his last combat (*Il.*, XXII, 105). Thirst for honor and fame, obverse sides of one and the same disposition of the soul, and the fear of public reproach are the principal motives of the powerful moral strength of Homeric man.[2] It is true that both continue in force in the Greek cities: the Homeric idea of virtue (*aretê*) and of individual excellence (*kalokagathia*) does not die out in the ages of Solon and Pericles. But alongside and within them a deep sense of religious and moral guilt, only rarely and faintly perceptible in the *Iliad* and the *Odyssey*, progressively gains ground and strength throughout the Hellenic world, especially in continental Greece. Hesiod, Solon, Theognis, Aeschylus, and Herodotus (the last a Greek from the colonies) contain literary testimony of this profound change of position and sensitivity.

A detailed portrayal of this new position of Greek civilization would go far beyond the limits of my present task. I must forego it.[3] But I consider that the proper development of my inquiry calls for a rapid sketch of its twofold background. Firstly, my explanation must stand out against the background of the general attitude adopted by the Greek people toward the fact of disease throughout the archaic period of Hellenic culture;[4] secondly, both my particular account and this idea

---

the "point of honor"). The "pudor" (*shame, aidos*) to which Dodds here refers pertains to social standing.

2. See W. Jaeger, *Paideia, 1,* 1.

3. Those who wish more information—in addition to E. Rohde's *Psyche* (Spanish translation, Mexico, 1948), and the previously mentioned bibliography—may read *Vom Mythos zum Logos*, by W. Nestle (Stuttgart, 1940); *Griechentum,* by W. Kranz (Baden-Baden and Stuttgart), a book in which two other works of the author are included, *Kultur der Griechen* and *Griechische Literaturgeschichte,* as well as F. M. Cornford's studies *From Religion to Philosophy* (London, 1912), which is still valid despite its date, and *Principium Sapientiae. The Origins of Greek Philosophical Thought* (Cambridge, 1952).

4. With Dodds and almost all present-day Hellenists I call the "archaic period" of Greek culture that contained between the "Homeric" and "classic" periods. It is part of what F. G. Welcker termed the "Middle Age" of Hellenic history.

of human illness require, in order to be understandable and understood, an adequate definition of their relative position within the life to which they belonged, or at least within the patterns of that life which were closest to them. Let us begin by pointing out the latter.

Here the religious, moral, and psychological ingredients of the guilt culture that established itself in Greece beginning in the seventh century B.C. are particularly important. In the matter of religion men's attitude toward the Divinity undergoes a perceptible change; mortal men, even under the deep fear of committing the sin of *hubris*, or excess, feel more heavily the influence the immortal gods bring to bear upon their fate. A famous phrase of Herodotus about the gods—"jealous and trouble-makers," he calls them—very strongly expresses the new situation of men's souls. Among the Hellenic people, for another thing, forms of religious belief different from the Olympic faith appear and spread to reveal those longings for immortality, happiness, and freedom in the afterlife that beat obscurely in the hearts of the post-Homeric Greek; it will suffice to mention the orgiastic cult of Dionysus, the Orphic and Eleusinian mysteries, and the worship of Cybele by the Corybantes. Dionysus, Orpheus, Cybele, and the divinities of Eleusis performed for their worshippers both a liberating and a purifying function. Finally, the considerable frequency with which *daimônes*, sometimes kindly, usually malign, are mentioned in the literary texts of the period must be noted. The consciousness of being "interfered with" by an unknown power from without—bear in mind that the *daimôn* began its existence in Hellenic culture—grows perceptibly among the Greeks following Homer's time. Perhaps it may be sufficient to observe, among the multitude of possible examples, that Theognis does not hesitate to call fear and hope "dangerous *daimônes*." In the Greece of Solon and Aeschylus man feels the silent threat of the unknown constantly about him.

Intimately connected with this change in religious attitude is another, touching on the moral life, whose center is the vague and diffuse sense of guilt previously mentioned. The blinding, impassioned fury that the Greeks called *atê* ceases to be an unforeseeable psychic accident and is changed into a punishment or calamity: Theognis calls the misfortune of receiving counterfeit gold *atê* (I, 119); for Euripides, Antigone and Ismene are the *atai* of Creon (*Tro.*, 530). The importance and the extent that cathartic rites attain in Greece, both in public life as well as in individual and private existence, make this general guilt-consciousness very evident. However summary my sketch, mention of the significant and famous "purification" of Athens by the purger Epimenides of Crete toward the end of the seventh century is necessary here. The punitive contamination of human reality and of cosmic reality by an invisible *miasma*—it is not infrequent for the *miasma* to be known as a *daimôn*—now is transformed into an ominous and constant possibility. Not even rectitude in personal behavior affords freedom from guilt and punishment, for to Hellenic eyes the contaminating "stain" comes to be not only contagious but also hereditary. The personal fate of individuals belonging to tragic lineages (the Atridae of Argos, the Labdacidae of Thebes) well illustrates the common Hellenic belief in this hereditary, and finally "physical," character of moral impurity.[5] It cannot be surprising that in the cities there were swarms of the professional purgers to whom Plato alludes in a famous passage of the *Republic:* "the charlatans and soothsayers who go about knocking at the doors of the rich and who convince them that they have received from the gods the power to cancel, by means of conjurations performed amid merriment and feasts, any fault that any of them or of their ancestors may have committed" (*Rep.*, II, 364b). Not only does *katharsis* become more frequent in post-Homeric Greece; also, and this is even more significant, it is professionalized and passes into the hands of persons specializing in the paid performance of purifying rites.[6]

That deep sense of guilt necessarily had to manifest itself in

---

5. Recall what was said in the previous chapter.
6. Regarding the probable Orphic status of those professional cath-artists whom Plato vilifies, see Boyancé, *Le culte des Muses chez les philosophes grecs* (Paris, 1937), pp. 11 ff.

the mind of Hellenic man. Together with the fear of the sin of *hubris* and moral impurity, the psychic powers of "irrational" nature and the types of behavior that correspond to them had continued to gain importance in Greek minds. The *mania*, the ecstatic rapture caused by the gods—a pathological rapture in madness and epilepsy, an ennobling and beneficent rapture in the forms of divine possession which Plato describes in the *Phaedrus* [7]—is not mentioned in the Homeric epic, unless it be in a very vague and precarious way.[8] In eloquent contrast to that silence, Herodotus, the tragedians, Empedocles, the *Corpus Hippocraticum*, and Plato attest to the frequency with which the Greek people bore in mind the psychological reality of the *theia mania* during the centuries following the eighth. And the growing importance attributed to dreams in Greece during that same period of her history has a quite parallel significance.[9]

What were the causes by virtue of which the "shame culture" presented to us in the epic came to be a "guilt culture"?

7. Those forms are four: the prophetic *mania* in which Apollo places the Pythoness of Delphi, the telestic or ritual *mania* of the worship of Dionysus, the poetic *mania* inspired by the Muses, and the erotic *mania* that Aphrodite and Eros bestow upon men and animals (*Phaedrus*, 244–265b).

8. Dodds (p. 67) can cite only two passages of the *Odyssey*. When Ulysses presents himself in the palace of Ithaca in disguise and the slave Melanthus calls him *ekpepatagmenos*, "out of his wits" (*Od.*, XVIII, 327), it is probable that this means merely what we do when we say that someone is "a little touched," although Dodds thinks that such an expression originally might have alluded to demonic interference. A little later (*Od.*, XX, 377) one of the suitors refers to Ulysses calling him *epimaston alêtên*. In contrast to the usual translation of *epimastos*, "beggar," Dodds thinks that this word comes from *epimainomai* and means "mad" or "touched." The author of *The Greeks and the Irrational* may well be right. As I have already said in the previous chapter, however, I do not believe that he is correct when he proposes to interpret as madness the "illness" that, in the opinion of the Cyclops, Zeus had sent Polyphemus (*Od.*, IX, 410 ff).

9. See J. S. Lincoln, *The Dream in Primitive Cultures* (London, 1935); J. Hundt, *Der Traumglaube bei Homer* (Greifswald, 1935); Ad. Palm, *Studien der Hippokratischen Schrift "Peri diaitês"* (Tübingen, 1933); Dodds, pp. 102–34; and P. Meseguer, *El secreto de los sueños* Madrid, 1956), as well as the bibliography on Asclepius given later.

And above all: was the real intensity of that change in Hellenic mentality as marked as literary sources lead us to believe? May it in fact be supposed that Homer, more concerned with the nobility of the epic genre than with documentary faithfulness of portrayal, and on the other hand deliberately confined within the latter to the ways of living peculiar to the Achaean aristocracy, stylized his description and omitted from it beliefs, sentiments, and practices then more frequent among the common people than among the nobles? Something of this must have occurred, according to the opinion dominant today among philologists who best know how to read the hexameters of the *Iliad* and the *Odyssey*. But a rapid comparison of the two poems suffices to show that in the *Odyssey* (chronologically the later) the passages in which that feeling of insecurity and guilt is revealed are more frequent. There is no doubt: the change in Greek mentality was real and intense. Even admitting the involuntary, selective stylization of Homeric description, the strong contrast between a poem of Homer and a tragedy of Aeschylus in regard to the reality and the idea of life that either presupposes makes it impossible to lessen the importance of the historic change that took place between the eighth and the fifth centuries. Using Nietzsche's very well-known antithesis, it is necessary to say that if the Homeric world was not purely "Apollonian," and if the tragic world in turn was not purely "Dionysian," the clear and powerful qualitative difference between them that the foregoing pages reveal did not therefore cease to exist. The problem consists in ascertaining the causes that determined such a difference.

According to present knowledge of the Greek Middle Age there appear to be two such causes. One regards Hellenic culture as a whole; the other pertains to life within the family. The social disorder following the Doric invasion—insecurity of the life of the individual, pessimism, sudden changes of economic and political character, overpopulation of continental Greece—is being accurately and topically brought forward by historians. With the establishment of the *polis*, the rise of democracy, and the transformation of the agricultural economy into a commercial and money economy, there rise to the surface of the social body forms of religiosity and of life formerly dominated by the old aristocracy and, above all, a spiritual climate arises favorable both to the intensification of certain ancient beliefs and to the spreading of others: orgiastic cults, Orphism, mysteries, the influence of *daimônes*, various magic rites. Magic arose from the sense of insecurity, according to Malinowski. To escape the threat that surrounded him the ancient Greek must have taken refuge in the irrational.

To this explanation of the change that occurred in post-Hellenic culture—an explanation very generally accepted and to which little objection can be made—Dodds has added another, compatible with it and more directly related to the genesis of the sense of guilt. In the strongly patriarchal Greek family of Homeric times the father is king and the son has no rights. The duty to honor and obey the father comes immediately after the duties to the gods (Pindar, *Pit.*, VI, 23–28), and Zeus himself rules on Olympus precisely because he is God the Father. Paternity and authority were intermingled in Homer's Greece and continued to be intermingled in the Greece of following centuries.

But could this patriarchal solidarity of the Greek family continue unaltered through the social crisis mentioned above? Undoubtedly not. With the establishment of the *polis* and the progress of democracy psychological tensions constantly arise within family life: the son feels in his heart a deep need for autonomy, and the father finds himself obliged to replace the old maxim, "you will do this because I say so," with "you will do this because it is right." A whole series of events—the juridical reform by Solon, the significant attitude of the Greeks to the myth of Cronos and Uranus, the frequency with which the dream of Oedipus is enacted in the fifth century among the Greeks (Sophocles, *Oed. R.*, 980–83; Herodotus, *Hist.*, VI, 107; Plato, *Rep.*, IX, 571c)—attest to that deep-seated and gradual transformation of family relations. It can now be understood why in Nephelococcygia or Cloud-cuckoo-land, the country of the Aristophanic utopia of the *Birds,* the rebellion of the son against the father is an admirable and applauded thing. It is not hard to detect the social and pedagogical reality of the sophistic movement under the winged and melodious jests of Aristophanes.

Present-day sociology, ethnology, and psychology allow one to suspect what took place in the souls of young Greeks during the seventh and sixth centuries. Psychologically, those souls must have experienced with deep inner vexation the ambivalence between the strong moral and affective bondage to patriarchal custom and a growing desire for independent existence, a desire which, as we have just seen, remained almost always unsatisfied until the second half of the fifth century. The genesis of the sense of guilt, subsequent almost always, as we know, to poorly repressed and sublimated desires, was thus almost inevitable. Greek life and mentality being what they really were, could that ambivalent vexation of soul persist without religious expression? The secret rebellion of son against father also becomes rebellion against Zeus, the heavenly Father and supreme key of cosmic order, and the sense of moral guilt is at the same time a sense of religious guilt. Attitudes of mind underlying the most characteristic words of Hellenic guilt culture necessarily must have prospered and spread in such a society: *hubris, miasma, katharsis, daimôn, mania, enthousiasmos, teletai.*[10]

Deep within this religious and moral world, before Pythagoras and Alcmeon of Crotona, Greek medicine was progressively taking shape. Taking for granted the existence of a grossly empirical medical practice—that employed by those who later are called, and perhaps were already called at that time, "rhizotomists" and "pharmacopolists," that which the successors of Nestor and Patroclus utilized in the treatment of wounds—I believe that the popular medicine of the Greek Middle Age can be described by distinguishing in it three principal traits:

1. Belief in the punitive character of disease becomes inten-

---

10. Only the last of these words requires translation: *teletai* were the religious ceremonies of those initiated into a religion of mysteries. See in this connection the discussion by P. Boyancé, pp. 11–31.

sified and widespread. The vague sense of guilt to which I have so often referred gave abundant encouragement to that process. Disease, the punishment of a personal fault, of a collective transgression, or of a crime of one's ancestors (Aeschylus, *Coeph.*, 278–81; *Suppl.*, 262–70; Sophocles, *Oed. R.*, 96–99; Plato, *Phaedrus*, 244 a e), was popularly conceived of as the contamination of the individual "nature" of the patient by a more or less invisible *miasma* or as the possession of the patient either by a god having a name (Hecate, Cybele, Pan, and the Corybantes, according to Euripides, *Hippol.*, 141 ff.; Hecate, Cybele, Poseidon, Enodia, Apollo Nomios, Ares, and the Heroes, according to the enumeration in the work *de morbo sacro*, Littré, 6, 360–62), or by an anonymous divinity, an obscure malign *daimôn* (Euripides, *Med.*, 129–30; *Hippol.*, 241; the pseudo-Hippocratic work *de virginibus*, Littré, 8, 466). What it expresses and what was said then specifically about epilepsy and madness must have been no less said of any disease of sudden appearance and obscure and unknown etiology.[11]

2. As a psychosomatic consequence of the sense of guilt and of the rites to which this sense led, there appeared among the Greeks new "diseases" or at least states and accidents of the soul and body very close to what we call disease. The epidemic spread of the Dionysiac cult, writes Rohde, "left in the nature of Greek man a morbid inclination, a tendency to experience sudden and fleeting disturbances of his normal capacity to perceive and feel. Isolated pieces of information tell us of attacks of that transitory delirium, which affected whole cities in epidemic form." [12] Using present-day medical terminology rather broadly, it does not seem too venturesome to call the psychic life of the Greeks during their Middle Ages neurotic. "The line that separates perfect health from illness," Aeschylus was to say, "is extremely thin; for illness, her next-door neighbor, intermingles with her" (*Agam.*, 1001–03).

11. Regarding nonphysiological conceptions of disease, see L. Edelstein, "Greek Medicine in Its Relations to Religion and Magic," *Bulletin of the Institute of the History of Medicine,* 5 (1937), 201–46.
12. *Psyche,* chap. 9 (2), "La religión dionisíaca en Grecia."

3. In the treatment of diseases, magical cures of mantic or purificatory character become much more frequent: various enchantments, cathartic ceremonies, medical oracles, orgiastic cults, Asclepian temple sleep. A more or less efficacious empiricism and a magico-religious medicine were the two principal resources of the Greek people against disease during the centuries immediately prior to the establishment of pre-Socratic *physiologia*.[13]

4. According to all this, in Greek society of the eighth to the sixth centuries the physician was simultaneously a liberator from or purifier of the physical stain in which the disease seemed to consist (a "cathartist" more or less near to one or another religious cult) and an heir of some one of the "first discoverers" to whom the source of medical knowledge used to be popularly and mystically referred (an "expert" in the use of herbs and remedies).[14] It is no accident that Apollo and the

---

13. For all these forms of Greek medicine of religious and popular character—"belief" medicine, according to the terminology I have suggested elsewhere (*Historia de la Medicina moderna y contemporánea*, Barcelona, 1954)—see my *Introducción al estudio de la patología psicosomática*, already mentioned. To the bibliography listed therein should be added the previously cited books by Pfister, Boyancé, Dodds, and Moulinier. H. W. Parke and D. F. W. Wormell have recently devoted an important work to the oracle of Delphi (*The Delphic Oracle, 1–2*, Oxford, 1956). Since the investigations of O. Weinreich ("Antike Heilungswunder," *R.G.V.V.*, 8, 1, 1909), S. Herrlich (*Antike Wunderkuren*, Wiss. Beilage z. Jahresber. des Humboldt-Gymnasiums zu Berlin, 1911), and R. Herzog ("Wunderheilungen: Die Wunderheilungen von Epidaurus," *Philologus, Suppl. Bd. 22*, 1931), the historical and medical aspects of the worship of Asclepius have been masterfully studied by E. J. and L. Edelstein (*Asclepius. A Collection and Interpretation of the Testimonies, 1–2*, Baltimore, 1945, and K. Kerény (*Der göttliche Arzt*, Darmstadt, 1956).

14. On the interesting theme of the "first discoverers" see A. Kleingünter's "*Prôtos heuretês*. Untersuchungen zur Geschichte einer Fragestellung," *Philologus, Suppl. Bd. 26*, 1933. Aeschylus attributes the source of Greek medicine to Prometheus (*Prom.*, 478–83) and to Apis (*Suppl.*, 262–70). In regard to the Centaur Chiron, I refer the reader to F. G. Welcker ("*Epode oder die Besprechung*," pp. 3 ff), W. A. Jayne (*The Healing Gods of Ancient Civilizations*, 1925), Edelstein (*Asclepius, 2*), Kerény, and J. Rof Carballo (*El Centauro Quirón*, Madrid, 1957). In the work *de prisca medicina* one reads that the "first discoverers" (*prôtoi eurontes*) of the medical art, aware of their great discovery, judged that such an art "would deserve to be attributed to a god, as it is the custom to believe" (Littré, *1*, 600–02). See my study, "El escrito *de prisca*

ancient physicians are called *iatromantes* (Aeschylus, *Eum.*, 62–63; *Suppl.*, 263), nor that this word should come to be used metaphorically to express the "purifying" action of pain. "To teach old age itself, chains and hunger are the *iatromantes* of hearts, *phrenôn iatromanteis*," Aeschylus says on one occasion (*Agam.*, 1621–23). The shamanistic status of these *iatromantes* (Abaris, Apis, and Mopsus among the legendary ones; Onomacritus, Epimenides, and Zamolxis among those who became historical figures) and their connection with Orphism and the Dionysiac cults seems today more than probable. Pythagoras himself must have belonged to such a line of Greek shamans, however harsh the assertion may appear to many.[15]

Against this twofold background—the culture of the Hellenic Middle Ages and the idea of disease and medical practice in that period of Greek history—we shall study in this chapter the therapeutic use of the word, from the poems of Homer to the Platonic dialogues. In an initial section we shall consider the testimony of the lyric and tragic poets; later, in another, we shall try to explore the writings of the pre-Socratic philosophers and the Sophists. The attitude of the Hippocratic physician to therapy with the word will be the object of a special chapter, following that devoted to the work of Plato.

II. It hardly seems necessary to state, after all that has been said, that the charm or conjuration (*epôdê*) was widely used for the treatment of disease throughout the centuries between

---

medicina y su valor historiográfico," *Emérita*, *12* (1944), 1–28. All this seems formally to oppose the thesis of L. Englert ("Untersuchungen zu Galens Schrift Trasybulos," *Studien zur Gesch. der Med.*, Heft 18, Leipzig, 1929), according to which the origin of medicine was interpreted by the Greeks as a dilemma, *either* by mythological attribution to a god, *or* by a rationalistic hypothesis.

15. Regarding the problem of the *iatromantes* of Greek shamanism and of shamanism in general see, together with the books of Rohde, Boyancé, Dodds, and Mircea Eliade already indicated, the revealing work "Scythica," by K. Meuli in *Hermes*, *70* (1935), 137 ff. The "charlatans and soothsayers" of whom Plato speaks in the *Republic* (II, 364b) and the quacks that the author of the work, *de morbo sacro*, vilifies and combats do not seem to differ much from those legendary *iatromantes*.

the Homeric epic and Plato. I shall not repeat here what was said in the preceding chapter regarding the *epaoidê* of the sons of Autolycus and its more than likely ethnological and historical roots in the customs of the primitive peoples who by their fusion gave birth to Greece. Wherever the magic attitude of mind reigns or survives, incantation is used, and not only with medicinal intent. The use of the Greek *epôdê*, accordingly, stubbornly endures throughout the whole of Hellenic history, from Homer to the Byzantine world.

But despite that unbroken and monotonous survival of the *epôdê* and the very well-known resistance to change which popular or intrahistorical customs usually present, it is possible to discover within Greek culture the existence of a true "history" of incantation. The concrete reality of the latter receives its form and its content within the historical situation to which it belongs; therefore, although the magical intent of the charmer passes almost unchanged from one century to another, the form and the ingredients of the rite do not fail to undergo some degree of change with the passage of time. With respect to the *epôdê* mentioned in the *Odyssey* everything that we know today has been said. Something more can be said of the incantations used in post-Homeric Greece, and that is what I propose to undertake in this chapter.

Four main elements seem to determine the form of the Greek *epôdê* between Homer and Plato: Orphism, the cult of Dionysus, the art of divination of Delphi, and the mythical and firmly based prestige, from a religious point of view, that the poems of Homer and Hesiod acquire.

Since the publication of Meuli's paper and the books by Nilsson, Boyancé, Dodds, and Guthrie,[16] the Thracian Orpheus appears to our eyes as a master shaman of shamans. The founder of Orphism, a religious movement so decisive in the history of Greek culture, was at once wizard, enchanter, musician, and cathartist or purifier. A passage from Empedo-

---

16. W. K. C. Guthrie, *Orphée et la religion grecque* (French translation, Paris, 1956). The studies of Meuli, Nilsson, Boyancé, and Dodds have been cited previously.

cles on the transmigration of souls significantly associates soothsayers, minstrels, and physicians.[17] Accordingly, then Orpheus combined in himself the virtue of those three activities, a virtue which in ancient Greece carried with it also that belonging specifically to the wizard and the cathartist. Despite the effort of some philologists to distinguish two Orphisms, one noble and pure, that of the Orphic communities, and another degenerate, that of certain conjurers, cathartists, and wandering quacks (the Orpheotelestes and Mêtragyrtes, the "charlatans and soothsayers" of whom Plato will speak in the *Republic*) it is almost certain that there was no such division among the primitive followers of Orpheus, and that within Greek society all of them individually carried out the various shamanistic activities of their founder.

Let us now keep to our subject and try to fathom the structure of the Orphic enchantments. The most pertinent legend and the most ancient graphic depictions—among them, a Boeotian goblet of the latter part of the sixth century B.C.—show us Orpheus taming birds and beasts with the music of his lyre. Are we therefore to conclude that music and music alone was the agent of Orpheus' magic power? Or put in another way: did the word lack importance in the first Orphic enchantments?

The reply must be in the negative. Simonides of Ceos (frag. 27 Diehl) already attributes the magic power of Orpheus to song, and when Aeschylus, through the mouth of Aegisthus, contrasts the enchanting might of the Thracian wizard with the dullness of the Coryphaeus, he speaks expressly of the latter's words and of the former's tongue and voice (*Agam.*, 1628–30). "The fame of Orpheus as a great singer," Nilsson has written, "is not based upon his music but upon the poems he declaimed while accompanying himself on the lyre."[18] In short: the operative formula of Orpheus' magic charms was the charm, the *epôdê*, in the most literal and etymological

---

17. Diels, *Fragmente der Vorsokratiker*, 5th ed. (Berlin, 1934), B 146, 1.

18. *Geschichte der griechischen Religion*, 1, 654.

sense of the word: *epi-ôdê, in-cantamentum.* Moreover, from the point of view of the intention with which they were originally sung, the Orphic hymns must be considered as genuine *epôdai*. In a brilliant study of the relationship between music and magic, Combarieu was able to reach the following conclusion: "Magic formulas have passed through the following phases: at first they were sung; then they were recited; finally they were written upon a material object worn in some cases as an amulet." [19] All the forms of the Greek *epôdê* are included in this outline.

What were the purposes of the Orphic charm? How was the magical treatment of human disease ranked among them? Were magic charms, *epôdai*, employed in other medical-religious sects more or less close to Orphism? What role did the word play in these from a medical point of view? Before answering this list of questions let us look at the pre-Platonic texts in which *epôdai* are mentioned.[20]

After the *Odyssey* Pindar is the first to use the term *epaoidê*, still in an uncontracted form. The magic charm, the *epaoidê*, serves on one occasion in his odes as a love incantation and is named in significant connection with *mania* (frenzy): Aphrodite "first brought to men the bird of *mania* [*mania d'ornin*] and taught Jason's skillful son charms and formulas so that he could make Medea forget respect for her parents" (*Pyth.*, IV, 216-19). But Pindar is also acquainted with the medicinal use of the *epaoidê*. In the Third Pythian the poet sets forth the healing power of Asclepius and his training by the Centaur Chiron:

> Is it not he—Chiron—who of old taught the sweet artisan of robust health, Asclepius, the hero and healer of all ailments? . . . Apollo took him to the Centaur of Magnesia and committed him to his care, so that the latter might teach him to cure the dolorous ailments of men. To all those who come to him with ulcers arising in their flesh,

19. Combarieu, *La musique et la magie* (Paris, 1909).
20. Texts pertaining to the pre-Socratic thinkers and to the Sophists will be considered in the following section, as I have noted.

wounded in some part by the gleaming bronze or by the stone of the sling, with body injured by the heat of the summer or the cold of the winter, he frees them their ill, either by curing them with gentle charms or by applying to their limbs all kinds of medicaments or, finally, putting them on their feet by means of incisions. (*Pyth.*, III, 5–8 and 45–53)

In relation to our subject, leaving aside commentary on the etiological and therapeutical ideas which those verses contain, the principal questions that Pindar's famous text poses to us are: 1. With respect to the singer of Thebes, of what can those gentle charms of which he tells have consisted? 2. Since Asclepius learned from Chiron how to cure by means of charms, is the word then likely to play an important role in the medical treatments of the temples of Asclepius?

Further on I shall try to reply to this second question. The first has been raised by L. Edelstein: relating those two words of Pindar with a passage from the *Attic Nights* of Aulus Gellius he thinks that the Greek expression *malakais epaoidais* is literally translated by the Latin expression *modulis lenibus* ("with soft cadences"), and that it should be interpreted in this way. "When the pains of sciatica are most intense, they become diminished if a flute-player plays soft cadences," Aulus Gellius says he has read in the work *peri enthousiasmou* by Theophrastus. The role of music thus seems dominant in the *epaoidai* of Asclepius; these must have been natural melotherapy rather than magical logotherapy.

Can this interpretation be accepted? I do not think so. It seems beyond doubt that music had considerable importance in the Greek *epôdai*, particularly in the primitive ones. But both the comparison of this text of Pindar with the two others in which the poet uses the word *epaoidê*—the verse already mentioned (*Pyth.*, IV, 218) and the one from *The Nemean Odes*, VIII, 49, on which I shall comment later—and, on the other hand, the history of what the *epôdê* later became in

Greek culture makes it necessary to recognize the outstanding role of the word in the health-bestowing *epaoidai* of Asclepius. In Pindar's mind the gentle charms which the Centaur Chiron taught Asclepius could be no other than magic songs, songs in which the words, the verbal formula of the *epaoidê*, were to possess as much importance as the music, perhaps even more. In regard to diseases the magical procedure of the singers Chiron and Asclepius must not have differed greatly from that which we have seen Orpheus, the master of song and incantation, follow.

In the works and fragments which have come down to us Aeschylus uses no less than four times the terms *epôdê* and *epaeidê* (*Agam.*, 1021), both in their clearest and fullest magic sense.[21] Two of these (*Agam.*, 1021; *Eum.*, 649) express the irrevocable character of death: "When the dust has drunk a man's blood, once he has died," says Apollo in *Eumenides*, 647–49, "there is no resurrection for him. My father has invented no charms for this." Again, through the mouth of Clytemnestra, Aeschylus calls Agamemnon an *epôdos*, enchanter or charmer, who sacrificed his daughter on the shores of Aulis to obtain favorable winds on his way to Troy (*Agam.*, 1418). The sacrifice of Iphigenia must have had, accordingly, the value and signification of a magic *epôdê*. Finally, a brief, isolated fragment (Pap. Ox., 2.256, 9a: 20) seems to tell us that the author opposes to the efficacy of a certain device the magical power of the charm.

Sophocles is more moderate and circumspect. In the *Trachinianae* Heracles rejects the existence of an enchanter or charmer able to cure him without the aid of Zeus: "What enchanter [*aoidos*], what artificer of healing [*cheirotechnês iatorias*], shall enchant, without Zeus, the ill that is killing me?" (*Trach.*, 1001–03). Sophocles seems to be establishing here a contrast between the wizard who tries to cure with charms and the physician who uses his hands to treat the patient—a contrast even more evident when Ajax, a little before

21. Regarding the nonmagical senses of the term *epôdê*, see my comments below.

taking his own life, casts into the air the famous cry: "It is not fitting for wise physicians to recite charms [*epôdas*] in the case of ailments that demand the knife" (*Ajax*, 581–82). The great tragedian still does not reject in an absolute fashion the use of *epôdai* for therapeutic purposes, but he already knows that there are diseases against which charms have no power, and he does not admit the reality of magical acts which have not been well tested by experience. A dialogue in the *Trachiniae* between Deinaria and the Coryphaeus speaks most eloquently: "My faith," says Deinaria, referring to the supposed magic power of Nessus' tunic, "is but a presumption; I have not put it to the test"; and the Coryphaeus replies, "It is necessary to know by experience, for even believing in success, you cannot be certain unless you have attempted it" (*Trach.*, 590–93). Such a prudent way of thinking was not very far from the critical spirit that Anaxagoras and the Sophists were able to create among the people of Athens.

The characters of Euripides, too, continue to give testimony of the popular use of the charm and show very clearly the connection between incantations and Orphism. In the *Cyclops* the Coryphaeus says that he is acquainted with an "excellent charm [*epôdê*] of Orpheus" to finish off Polyphemus. Ulysses' reply is very significant. He rejects the magic means offered him, but he immediately thereafter allows the "melodious songs" of the satyr to lend courage to his friends (*Cycl.*, 646–53). If Euripides' "enlightened" Ulysses no longer believes in the power of magical incantations he nevertheless does not disdain the strengthening effect of songs. The enchanting power of the words of Orpheus is mentioned twice in *Alcestis:* the magic words are in one case "hymns" (359) and in another signs written upon some "Thracian tablets." Against Necessity or *Anankê*—in this instance, in regard to the death of Alcestis—nothing can be done, says the chorus: "I, by dint of association with the Muses, darted to heaven, and among many reasons which I observed, I found none stronger than Necessity, nor is there any remedy against her in the Thracian tablets which the melodious Orpheus inscribed, nor in all the chosen medicaments which Phoebus gave the followers of Asclepius for mortal victims of disease" (*Alc.*, 965–72).[22] And Iphigenia too thinks of the incantations of Orpheus when, powerless before her tragic fate, she dreams of possessing the magic power which she does not have: "If I, oh my father, had Orpheus' language to persuade rocks with my charms [*peithein epadousa*], and make them follow me, and to bewitch [*kêlein*] with my words whomever I wished" (*Iph. Aul.*, 1211–13). Also the nurse of Phaedra and the nurse of Medea —in the tragedy the common people, with their traditional wisdom, their common sense, and their superstitious beliefs, always speak through nurses—have faith in the magical efficacy of *epôdai*. "You are ill," the former says to her mistress. "Put an end to your ailment with some propitious remedy. There are charms [*epôdai*] and enchanting words [*logoi thelktêrioi*]; a remedy for your ailment will appear" (*Hippol.*, 477–79).[23] Less decisive is the nurse of Medea: neither with festive hymns nor with songs accompanied by the lyre (*polychordois ôdais*) can the sorrows of men be mitigated, she tells us, but for all this she does not cease to believe in the curative power of song: "Mortals," she adds, "would obtain benefit by curing through songs [*akeisthai molpaisi*]" (*Med.*, 195–203). The messenger in *The Phoenician Women* expresses an equal faith in the magic word when he says to Jocasta: "If you possess some recourse, if you know wise words [*sophous logous*] or bewitching charms [*philtr'epôdôn*], depart" (Phoen., 1259–60).

22. I follow A. Tovar's translation in *Eurípides, Tragedias, 1* (Barcelona, 1956), 76–77. In regard to the discussion of what those "Thracian tablets" might have been, see Boyancé, p. 39. As the scholiast observes, it is the author Euripides who is speaking here through the mouth of the chorus. In his edition for *Les Belles Lettres* (4th ed. Paris, 1956, pp. 93–94) Méridier points out that this passage from *Alcestis* shows the "enlightened" and philosophical character of Euripides.

23. Méridier comments: "This language is deliberately of double meaning. It may refer to charms and magical words suitable for *making love vanish*, as well as to utterances able to *satisfy it* by awakening the passion in the person who is the object of this love." The frequency of popular beliefs in the action of love potions inclines rather to the admission of the second hypothesis.

A brief phrase of Hecuba seems to place the supposed magical efficacy of the *epôdai* in connection with the evocative and evil-averting power of names rightly uttered. When Polymestor foretells to Hecuba that her tomb will be known by an epithet, she replies: "Called after my form [*Morphês epôdon*], or what else are you about to say?" (*Hec.*, 1272). The utterance of this epithet would be a charm evoking the form of Hecuba. More than a song, the *epôdê* is now an efficacious word, a verbal formula accurately known and uttered.[24]

Less clear is the magical action of dancing and song in *Electra*, despite the use of the verb *epaeidein* to designate that action (*El.*, 864). As to the *epôdos* that appears on one occasion in the *Bacchae* (234), the reader is referred to what is said at a later point in this study.[25]

The terms *thelktêrion* and *kêlêma* or *kêlêtêrion* possess by themselves a much broader meaning than *epôdê*; they mean "enchantment," "sorcery," or "bewitchment" in their most general sense. They are, accordingly, magical actions per-

24. Not far from this faith in the efficacy of the true name is a famous invocation of Zeus in Aeschylus' *Agamemnon*: "Zeus, whoever he may be, by this name I invoke him, if this name pleases him" (*Agam.*, 160–62). But A. Lesky sagaciously comments: "The most ancient cultural formula of the hymn of invocation is used here. Its ultimate root is the idea, widely spread throughout the whole world, of the magic power of the name: whoever wishes to reach the god with his invocation must call him by his true name, and if he has several by all of them. But what depth of content that ancestral form has received in Aeschylus! When he begins with the phrase *Zeus ostis pot'estin*, in that "Whoever he may be" he is not expressing a sophistic doubt about the possibility of knowing something about the divine being, but rather the fullness of his heart which no longer can name its god with words and, at the same time, the superiority of this god to that one to whom Homeric poetry had given the name of Zeus" (*Die griechische Tragödie*, 2d ed. Stuttgart, 1958, pp. 101–02).

25. Among Greek prose writers Herodotus is the first to have used the word *epaoidê*. When he describes the ritual sacrifices of the Persian magi, he states that the officiating priest sings a "theogony" (I, 132) as a sort of incantation (*epaeidei*). The priest, Pfister comments, "is here, accordingly, the *arêtêr*, the one who entreats, the only one who knows the truly efficacious words and who can utter them" (*RE* Suppl. Bd. 4, 321–27). Pausanias too (V, 27, 6) speaks of the *epôdai* of the Persian magi: "they sing a barbarous conjuration, incomprehensible to the Greeks, to a certain god," says the account.

formed by any of the procedures to which magicians resort, and not merely by means of the "songs" to which the expressions *epi-ôdê* and *in-cantamentum* etymologically and historically allude. But there are cases in which the former three terms as well—and like them the verbs from which they come, *thelgô* and *kêleô*, "enchant" and "bewitch"—name magical actions performed by means of the human word, actions, moreover, of therapeutic character. According to a fragment from Archilochus, "every man who lives is bewitched [*kêleitai*] by songs [*aoidais*]" (frags. 106 Diehl, 19 R. Adrados).[26] Is Archilochus speaking in a general sense of the enchanting joy that beautiful songs produce in the souls of those who listen to them, or is he referring to the magical enchantment of those that specifically possess such a power? Put otherwise: is the verb *kêleô*, "bewitch," used here in its proper meaning or in a metaphorical sense? It does not seem possible to decide with certainty. Less dubious may be the metaphorical intention of the Fourth *Nemea* of Pindar, where the poet declares that his songs (*aoidai*) will be able to enchant or bewitch (*thelxan*) the toils of harsh life: in the happiness (*euphrôsynê*) that the former produce the latter would find their best physician (*Nem.*, IV, 4–5). The rhetoric of Pindar's odes, the poetic word of the bard, acts accordingly by enchanting the minds of its hearers and effacing the inevitable pains of daily existence.

In tragedy the mention of *thelktêria* (charms) and *kêlêmata* (bewitchments) of verbal ritual is no less evident.[27] We shall soon have occasion to observe how the tragic authors allude to such rites, although in a metaphorical way. Here a brief cita-

---

26. I refer the reader to the excellent edition of the latter author, which in more than one respect is superior to Diehl's: *Líricos griegos. Elegíacos y yambógrafos arcaicos* (Ediciones Alma Mater, Barcelona, 1956).

27. Nonverbal types of *thelktêria*—or, at least, not explicitly verbal—are those mentioned by Aeschylus (*Suppl.*, 571: Zeus "enchants" the pain of Io, harassed by the gadfly; *Prom.*, 865: amorous enchantments of Aphrodite, etc.), Sophocles (*Trach.*, 355 and 585: bewitchment of Heracles), and Euripides (*Iph. Taur.*, 166: offerings to appease the dead; *Hippol.*, 509: potions to produce love by magic, etc.). The same can be said of *kêlêma* (Euripides, *Tro.*, 893; *Hec.*, 535, etc.).

tion of a passage from Aeschylus of clearly medical-moral sense may suffice. Determined to eradicate the curse and the hereditary stain that weighs heavily upon Orestes, Apollo promises him to free him forever from his sorrows by means of "enchanting tales" (*thelktêrious mythous*) (*Eum.*, 81–83). The word of Apollo enchants, purifies, and heals. Not in vain does Pindar declare (*Pyth.*, IV, 176) that the lineage of Orpheus, "father of songs," has its source in Apollo.

The semantic relationship of the three Greek words that designate "enchantment"—*epôdê, thelktêrion, kêlêma*—is, accordingly, quite evident. The practice of the *epôdê* almost always involved the use of magical songs, but at times enchantments that were not sung are designated by that name. But on the other hand *thelktêria* and *kêlêmata* in which music and words constitute the operative formula of the enchantment are not infrequent.[28] Hence it is that the questions that remained unanswered several pages back can be referred to these three magical concepts. For what purposes was the Orphic charm practiced? Within those purposes, how was the magic treatment of human disease ranked? Did the magic verbal charms have a place within the medical-religious sects more or less close to Orphism?

With one name or another, under one form or another, the Greek incantation sought the magical attainment of all that man needs and cannot obtain by means of his natural resources: favorable weather, love at will, the automatic obedience of another person, preternatural alteration of the cosmos, the cure of disease. Under the pressure of the charm the powers superior to man—gods with their own names or obscure and unnamed *daimônes*—would yield to the desire of the enchanter or of persons who had sincere recourse to him. But together with the apotropaic process—better expressed, as a result of it —another of cathartic nature was not uncommonly performed: the charm "purified" from defiling *miasmata* and *dai-*

---

28. A previously quoted verse of Euripides (*Alc.*, 359) calls the act of enchanting by means of Orphic hymns *kêlein*. As in so many other cases, this is an enchantment at once musical and verbal.

mônes the reality "enchanted" by it regardless of whether the latter was man, animal, or inanimate object. "Orpheus," Pausanias, expressing the feeling of the Greek people, would later say, "was much superior to his predecessors in the beauty of his song and came to have so much power that it is believed that he invented the initiation of the goddesses, the purifications of sacrileges, cures for diseases and means to avert the wrath of the gods." [29]

Alone or accompanied by music, the magic word sings to the gods in the ceremonies of the initiates (*teletai*), performs marvelous acts, among them, the curing of diseases, and purifies the impure. Does this mean that the power of the charm is judged to be omnipotent? We do not know with enough precision how far the belief of the Greek people may have extended during the centuries of its Archaic Age. But literary evidence of the fifth century expresses with great clarity the deep conviction that the magic power of enchantment is confined by impassible boundaries: the *moira* or fate of every man, Nature, Necessity. "Thou hast sought to enchant the unenchantable," says the chorus of the Danaides to their handmaidens in the *Suppliants* of Aeschylus (1056). For the daughters of Danaus there is something which, even above the designs of the gods, is unenchantable, *athelkton,* in this case the stubborn nuptial will of Aphrodite. And what other than *moira* could be the ultimate cause of this limitation? [30] Electra thinks the same of the sufferings that her cruel fate imposes upon her: "They can be mitigated, but not enchanted [*thelgetai*]," she says to the chorus (*Coeph.,* 420). Death, for its part, cannot yield to charms and is not magically revocable (*Agam.,* 1021; *Eum.,* 649); it obeys the inexorable law of Necessity or *Ananké* (Euripides, *Alc.,* 965). In other words: in

---

29. Pausanias, IX, 30, 4. I follow the translation by A. Tovar, *Pausanias. Descripción de Grecia,* University of Valladolid, 1946. Diodorus also (II, 29; III, 58) will place charms in relationship to "purifying agents" or *katharmoi.* For the relationship between *epôdê* and *katharsis* in the work of Plato see the following chapter.

30. For the role of *moira* in Greek thought see W. C. Greene, *Fate, Good and Evil in Greek Thought* (Cambridge, Mass., 1948).

nature there are necessary events against which the power of enchantments has no effect. And not only death—in certain cases disease and pain as well: "Ills such as mine have always been held incurable," says Sophocles' Electra (*El.*, 229–31). Experience—that *peira* to which, as we have already seen, the Coryphaeus of the *Trachiniae* knows how to appeal—will at length show enlightened Greeks the true power of the magic charm. But will the unenlightened Greeks cease to believe in it?

The orgiastic rites of the cult of Dionysus had in Hellenic eyes a potent curative power as well. One of the epithets of Dionysus is that of *Lysios* (liberator), and today it seems generally accepted that with this term an allusion was made to the healing character of the god: Dionysus, liberator from ills and particularly from madness and Bacchic frenzied rapture.[31] By means of the *enthousiasmos* of the ritual orgy and through a kind of psychic homeopathy the god purified and cured his faithful. He healed them directly of the madness with which he usually punished resistance to the acceptance of his cult (according to the legend, such was the case of the daughters of Minyas at Orchomenus and of the daughters of Proetus at Tiryns), and by extension he freed them from every possible disease. Directly supported in the cult of Dionysus the almost mythical medicaster Melampus worked with his spells and with "ineffable sacrifices and purifications" (Pausanias, VIII, 18, 6–7), and Pausanias attributes also to Dionysus the theurgical treatments of a priest of Amphiclea: "Very worthy to be seen [in Amphiclea] are the orgies of Dionysus . . . The ailments of the people of Amphiclea and their neighbors are cured by means of dreams, and the priest is a seer, who answers possessed by the god" (X, 23, 11).[32]

Now in those Dionysiac "cures" did the human word play any role or were music and the dance alone the means of its

---

31. See a brief report on ancient and modern discussion of the epithet *Lysios* in Boyancé, p. 16.
32. For everything bearing on the worship of Dionysus see the previously cited bibliography, especially the books of Rohde and Nilsson.

possible physical efficacy? "We have no knowledge of songs being sung in the worship of Dionysus," writes Rohde, "probably because the violence of the dance took away the breath of the celebrants and did not allow them to sing. But the rhythm of these orgiastic dances was not, to be sure, the gentle and measured cadence with which the Greeks of Homer moved to the sounds of the paean, but a sort of furious, delirious whirlwind that drove the throngs of dancers headlong over the hillsides like an overflowing river."[33] Pausanias, on the other hand, calls the purifying or cathartic rites of Melampus "ineffable" or "unspeakable" (*aporrêtoi*). We must conclude from this that in Dionysiac psychotherapy, if the term may be allowed, there were belief, cries, frenzied dancing, and music (brazen horns, tambourines, Phrygian flutes), but no "word" in the strict sense. Within the Nietzschean conception of the Dionysiac one could speak of therapy *aus dem Geiste der Musik*. And thus the reproach of *epôdos* or "charmer" that Euripides flings on one occasion at Dionysus (*Bac.*, 234) must be understood in its metaphoric sense of "magician" or "sorcerer," since the orgiastic cult had no place at all for the *epôdê* as a sung or recited charm.[34]

But if orgiastic psychotherapy had no verbal character, the contrary is certainly true of the oracles and exorcisms—often of therapeutic intent—of the ecstatic seers who in some particular sanctuary, such as that of Amphiclea mentioned by Pausanias, or wandering from one city to another like those who later would be called Bacchides and Sibyls, had some genetic connection with the Thracian god. This, without taking up the difficult problem of the relationship between Dionysus and

33. *Psyche*, chap 8 (2).
34. Exaggerating matters a bit, one might say that Dionysus was such an enemy of the word that he drove mad those who used it to argue against him. "The impetuous son of Dryas [Lycurgus] was also subjected to Necessity," it is stated in the *Antigone* of Sophocles, "who because of his violent fits of madness was confined by Dionysus in a stone prison. So the terrible, exuberant fury of his madness declined. He recognized that it was senseless to attack the god with insolent speeches, because he was seeking to put an end to the frenzy of the Bacchantes" (*Antig.*, 955–64).

Apollo, leads us to consider briefly the medical aspect of the oracles of Delphi and the cult of Apollo.

In the Homeric epic Apollo appears as a healing god. Although he was subsequently displaced from this function by his son Asclepius—let us not forget that Apollo was prior to Asclepius in the temple of Epidaurus—he never ceased to be invoked in the distressing crisis of illness. Many of the Greek epithets of the god—*akesios, epikouros, alexikakos*—allude to his physicianly character; *Apollo medicus* the Romans will continue to call him. Clement of Alexandria, Christianizing this old belief in Apollo's therapeutic efficacy, will not hesitate to call Christ the "paeonic physician" (*Paedag.*, I, 2, 6). But was this healing efficacy of Apollo only medicinal—Euripides speaks, as we already know, of "the chosen medicaments which Phoebus gave to the followers of Asclepius" (*Alc.*, 969)—or did it also make use of the word?

The reply must now be in the affirmative. Apollo, in fact, bequeathed to the Greeks two forms of the therapeutic word: the paean and the oracle. Let us recall the "beautiful paean" with which Ulysses and his comrades ask Apollo to end the plague that is decimating the Achaeans (*Il.*, 1, 473). That canticle doubtlessly had a beseeching intent. Only beseeching? Was Ulysses' paean *only* a prayer? Present-day philology and ethnology empower us to say something more.[35] *Paiêôn*, the name of the god who on Olympus cures Hades and Ares (*Il.*, V, 401 and 899–90), *Paiôn*, the epithet of Apollo as a healer, and *paian*, the paean or solemn song of beseechment or praise, are words etymologically and semantically related to one another. Accordingly, a detailed study of the texts in which those three words appear makes it possible to reconstruct the process of their indubitable semantic mutation. At an initial period *paiêôn* was a name given to magical songs of curative character. Many centuries later Proclus, taking up a last remnant of this very ancient Greek opinion, will say in his *Chres-*

---

35. L. Deubner, "Paian," *N. Jahrb. für klass. Alt.*, 43, 1919, 385 ff.; Nilsson, *Griechische Feste*, p. 100, and *Geschichte der Griechischen Religion*, *1*, 147–48 and 511–12.

tomathy that the paean is "a canticle for the ending of plagues and diseases." *Paiêôn*, the physician-god of Olympus, a god without autonomous existence and without his proper cult, must have been no more than a personification of those magical songs. Later the words *Paiêôn*, and *Paiôn* become epithets of the healer Apollo; written with a small *p* (*paiêôn, paiôn*) or changed into *paian* they will become nouns designating the religious canticles of praise to the god, of prayer and victory, until at last the term *paian*, now secularized, will serve to specify a literary form. Therapeutic magic, religious worship, and literary technique are accordingly the three principal stages in the history of the paean.[36] And this, which is now of special importance, leads us to the discovery that the paean of Ulysses in Book I of the *Iliad* and the *epaoidê* of the sons of Autolycus in Book XIX of the *Odyssey* are but two forms and two different names of the same rite: the rite of "enchanting" disease by magic songs. Through Apollo in the case of the paean, and probably also in the case of the *epaoidê*, the human word might have the magic power to heal mortal men. Invoked by Glaucus, Phoebus Apollo allays his pains, stanches the blood of his wound, and instills courage into his spirit (*Il.*, XVI, 527–28). This is what the Greeks will always expect of Apollo the Healer when they sing his paeans and *epôdai* or, once the practice of enchantment becomes "professionalized," when they charge others to aid them by magic to get out of their predicaments.

The verbal aspect of the healing power of Apollo is not limited to the paean; to it belongs the oracle as well. Inspired divination often had a therapeutic character. Faced with the plague of Thebes, Oedipus sends his brother-in-law Creon to Delphi so that the latter may "learn what he, Oedipus, must do or say to save the city" (*Oed. R.*, 69–72). "In their fits of madness," Plato will write, "the prophetess of Delphi and the priestesses of Dodona conferred many benefits, public and private, upon Greece. Among others, prophetic madness found

36. Many of the words with which human activity is expressed have a history similar to that of the paean.

deliverance from the most horrible ailments and woes which, as a result of ancient guilts, and without it being known whence they come, afflict some families" (*Phaedrus*, 244 a e). The seer, *mantis,* is at the same time a physician, *iatros;* hence those effecting cures through exorcisms and oracles were, since the time of those legendary personages, more or less related to Apollo, such as Apis and Abaris the Hyperborean, who enjoyed such high and ancient prestige in Greece and were called *iatromantes.* We now know that even Apollo himself could receive from Aeschylus the name of *iatromante* (*Eum.*, 62) because to him were attributed the curative oracles of Delphi and of so many other places in which he spoke as the god of good health.[37]

Did the mysteries of Eleusis have any relation to the treatment of disease? And if they had, was that relation of verbal character? The historians of Greek religion say very little about this and the historians of medicine even less. But if, as is recognized today, there was a real connection between Orphism and Eleusis, and if, as Boyancé thinks, this connection had its innermost strength in the idea of the magical incantation, it appears that the reply to these two questions must be in the affirmative. In fact the author of *Le culte des Muses* says:

> The mutual approach of enchantments and *teletai* (the religious ceremonies of initiation and of the initiate) is based upon a very important characteristic of these rites: both act upon the gods with a kind of irresistible action derived largely from the magic power of word and song. If Orpheus and the Orpheans are bound so closely to the mysteries, it is because they are the most eminent specialists in enchantment; accordingly, neither "Orphic life,"

---

37. Apollo gave health and could send or announce disease. To the plague of Book I of the *Iliad* may be added the "frightful diseases that attack the flesh and the leprosies that with fierce tooth devour a body hitherto sound," of which Orestes speaks (*Coeph.*, 278–81). "There is no physician who can provide a remedy for my prediction," the inspired Cassandra says for her part.

nor mere moral preaching is at the source of that bond, but something more primitive and perhaps more profound.[38]

In the rites of Eleusis there was not only silence and vision, there was also the word, *logos*. Ancient indeed are the accounts of the "secret words" (*aporrêta*) of the Eleusinian mysteries: rhythmic verbal formulas, reserved for the initiates, recited or sung by the hierophant and then repeated by the faithful. In the minds of those who pronounced them, did these mysterious *aporrêta* have some medicinal power of magic character? Nothing seems more likely. The judgment of Aristotle regarding the psychic state of those participating in the mysteries—that state "is not a perceiving [*mathein*], "says the philosopher, "but a passion [*pathein*] and a disposition of the spirit" (frag. 15 Rose)—strengthens the probability of this conjecture. From a medical point of view *aporrêta* and *teletai* in Eleusis were in all probability something very similar to what the hymns and Orphic *epôdai* and the paeans of the more primitive cult of Apollo were becoming in other parts of Greece.

There remains to be considered (leaving the examination of Pythagoreanism for the following chapter) the role of the word in the therapy of the Asclepian temples. Did those "gentle charms" that the son of Apollo learned from the Centaur Chiron, according to Pindar's account, play any role in the cures of Epidaurus and the other Asclepian sanctuaries? The usual description of sleep in the temple, beginning with the famous one by Aristophanes (*Pluto*, 633–747), calls for a completely negative reply: Asclepius did not cure in his temples by verbal formulas and songs of magic character; the words that the patient heard during his sleep in the temple—therefore while dreaming or in a half-dreaming state—were only those pertaining to the therapeutic description by the god. Only in a very few cases did those words have oracular character, and the content or the oracles of Asclepius was not always medical. Does this mean that verbal psychotherapy—

38. *Le culte des Muses*, p. 58.

nontechnical and unintentional psychotherapy, of course—was totally absent from the cures of Epidaurus? Not at all. A detailed examination of the sources brings to light psychotherapeutic features in the beneficent speech of Asclepius the Healer. At times the beauty and softness of his voice played their part—*emmelestaton phthongon,* a most "harmonious voice," according to an account of Suidas (*Lexicon,* under *Domninos*); *placido emittere pectore voces,* "he spoke with a peaceful spirit," is said in another account by Ovid (*Metam.,* XV, 657)—and at times what that voice communicated to the patient was equally effective. Oribasius relates that Asclepius appeared to Teucer of Cizicus during his incubation in the temple of Pergamum, conversed with him, and asked him if he wished his illness (Teucer suffered from epileptic seizures) to be exchanged for another (*Coll. Med.,* XLV, 30, 10–14); even more clear and eloquent is a report of Galen, according to which Asclepius not infrequently assigned to patients the task of composing odes, comic skits, and songs in order to correct the disproportion, or *ametria,* of the emotions in their soul (*de san. tuenda,* I, 8, 19–21). There is no doubt: without an expressly magic intention, but certainly directly based upon the deep faith of the Greek people in the curative power of Asclepius, his words often had an undeniably psychotherapeutic character.

What has been stated can now be summed up in this brief conclusion: under various names—*epôdê* or "charm," *thelktêrion* and *kêlêma* or "spell," *paiêôn* or "paean," *aporrêta* or "secret words," and *teletai* or "rites of initiation"[39]—against the painful event of human disease, archaic Greece made wide use of verbal formulas of magic character, merely recited at

---

39. To this list could be added the word *horkos,* "oath." In the preceding chapter, I indicated a passage in Aeschylus (*Agam.,* 1198–99) which reveals a belief in the curative and purificatory power of the oath. For the significance of the oath among the Greeks, see Wilamowitz, *Der Glaube der Hellenen, 1* (Berlin, 1931), 32. An analogous curative and purificatory action must have been accomplished by the "speaking" (*ti phônôn*) which Oedipus will utter to free Thebes from the plague if the oracle of Delphi bids him do so (*Oed. R.,* 72).

times, usually sung. The content of those formulas was highly varied: religious hymns with the prestige of Antiquity, fragments from Homer and Hesiod, brief exclamations, and even unintelligible words.[40] The Greek people, and not only the common rabble, believed in magic and had frequent recourse to it from pre-Homeric times to the end of the Hellenistic period, that is, throughout their entire history. The philosophy of Plato, Aristotle, and the Stoics will be powerless against that vigorous belief or with certain restrictions will continue to accept it. Let us earnestly affirm this reality against so many excessive idealizations of Hellenic culture. But, this said, it is necessary and urgent to warn that when the authors of the fifth century use the words *epôdê*, *thelktêrion*, and *kêlêma* they are not always alluding to rites or ceremonies of magic character. Little by little, from the lyric poets of the sixth century to Plato, the metaphoric use of those three terms insinuates itself—a literary event that, under its apparent insignificance, is to have important consequences in the history of Greek culture.

Metaphoric senses of the verb *thelgô* (charm, enchant) and the noun *thelktêrion* (spell) (recall the final part of the preceding chapter) are not infrequent in the Homeric epic. The amorous spell that the girdle of Aphrodite contains (*Il.*, XIV, 215) and that gives the words of Calypso (*Od.*, I, 57) and the song of the Sirens (*Od.*, XII, 40) their dangerous power no doubt possessed in Homer's mind the character that today we are accustomed to call "magic." But when we are told that Penelope knew how to "charm the soul" (*thelge de thymon*) of her suitors with sweet words (*Od.*, XVIII, 282) or that the bard Phemius enchanted the hearts of those who heard him with his "bewitching tales" (*thelktêria*) (*Od.*, I, 337), then the sense of such terms cannot be other than metaphorical, for neither the words of Penelope nor the tales of Phemius are magic charms in the strong sense of this

---

40. A passage from Aristotle (frag. 454; FHG, II, 188) states that on a certain occasion the following charm was used against the plague: "Go to the crows!" With this the plague was to have been "charmed." When the verbal psychotherapy of the Pythagoreans is discussed, this theme of the contents of the ancient *epôdai* will reappear.

expression. Accordingly what had already begun in the verses of the epic becomes intensified in the literature of the fifth century. For examples I shall limit myself to the works of Aeschylus. In the *Suppliants* the King of the Argives speaks thus: "a bewitching tale [*mythos thelktêrios*] can cure an ill that other words have caused, but to prevent the blood of the Argives from being shed sacrifices are necessary" (*Suppl.*, 446–48). The metaphoric use of the adjective *thelktêrios,* already very evident in the first part of the phrase, now gains doubled clarity from the contrast between the human naturalness of the "bewitching tale" and the sacral character and supernatural power of the "sacrifice." Equally clear is the metaphorical transposition in two passages of the *Eumenides*. "If you respect venerable Persuasion, if my words are for your heart sweetness and enchantment [*thelktêrion*], you will remain here," says Athena to the chorus of the Eumenides (*Eum.*, 885–86), to which the Coryphaeus of the latter replies shortly thereafter: "It seems to me that my animosity, now bewitched, is yielding" (900). In all these passages we are told that the word "bewitches," so as to emphasize the power of its persuasive effect on the mind of one who listens to it. Thus the expressions *thelktêrios logos* or *thelktêrios mythos* in such cases should be translated by "persuasive speech" rather than by "bewitching speech." [41]

The same occurs with the noun *epôdê* and with the verb *epadô*, "charm" and "to charm." Pindar, for example, on one occasion calls his poems charms or enchantments (*epaoidai*): "I am much pleased when I give a heroic feat the praise it deserves and with my charms [*epaoidais*] the athlete sees his weariness allayed" (*Nem.*, VIII, 49–50). The metaphorical play of Pindar's boast is evident: the poet esteems the invigorating and persuasive power of his odes so highly that he dares to call them *epaoidai,* charms, as if that power were really magical. "I shall not let myself be bewitched [*thelxei*] by the

---

41. Even when there is no reference to a verbal expression but to the gratification of the body the metaphorical use of *thelktêrion* in *Coeph.*, 670, is also evident.

honeyed charms [*epaoidaisin*] of Persuasion," says Prometheus in Aeschylus' tragedy (*Prom.*, 172–74). Nor is it here a matter of magic charms in the strict sense of the term, but of seductive words; nor is Pericles being called a "sorcerer" by Eupolis, when the latter humorously tries to praise most highly the great talent of the Athenian statesman for verbal seduction (*Dem.*, frag. 98 EDM). The same metaphor appears by the end of the fifth century on the lips of the noble daughter of Oedipus: "Others too have guilty children and rash hearts, but counseled by the charms [*epôdais*] of their friends they enchant [pacify: *expadontai*] their nature" (Sophocles, *Oed. Col.*, 1192–94). Lastly, Theseus calls Hippolytus a charmer (*epôdos*) and bewitcher (*goês*) when he believes that the latter is trying to deceive him with his words (*Hippol.*, 1038).

The metaphorical use of the terms *epôdê* and *thelktêrion* for the purpose of vigorously emphasizing the suggestive power of the human word is, then, a fairly general occurrence in the Greek literature of the fifth century, an occurrence which we shall again see confirmed in the next chapter when we examine the psychotherapeutic aspect of the work of the Sophist Gorgias. One question at once arises in the mind of the historian: does this metaphorical transposition have a deep meaning or is it merely a fortuitous stylistic accident? A slight acquaintance with what Greek culture was from the time of Homer on is sufficient to give a proper reply: *the idea and the decision to apply boldly and hyperbolically the term "epôdê" to the suggestive word, to every verbal expression able to persuade through what it is in itself, had as their causes the very high prestige that the social efficacy of speech always enjoyed among the Greeks and the growing importance that skillful speech progressively acquired in the democratic "poleis" of the sixth and fifth centuries.* Pindar, Aeschylus, Sophocles, Eupolis, Gorgias, and Euripides feel in their hearts and observe in their milieu that speaking—speaking well—is at once knowledge and power, to such a point that the good speaker is comparable to men endowed with magic powers, the *epôdoi* or charmers. The mythical excellence of Achilles' upbringing

(*Il.*, IX, 443) and the legendary prestige of the bard (*Od.*, VIII, 479–80) carry over clearly into the historical and social consciousness of the Greeks of the fifth century, and therefore —this was the sophistry—into intellectual reflection and methods of education.

The psychological basis of that efficacy of the word receives the name of "persuasion" (*peithô*). It is no accident that *Peithô*, Persuasion, came to attain among the Greeks a divine status. Homer does not mention her, despite the importance which the literary expression of the epic grants to the verb *peithein*, "to persuade." *Peithô*, "august Persuasion," appears as a goddess in the work of Hesiod: she is one of the daughters of Oceanus and Thetis (*Theog.*, 349) and is among the deities who adorn and make seductive the newly formed figure of Pandora (*Trab.*, 73). Later testimony (Ibycus, Sappho, Anacreon) presents her to us as a companion and aide of Aphrodite, and even (Aeschylus, *Suppl.*, 1041) goes so far as to declare her the latter's daughter. Peithô, according to this testimony, begins as the goddess of erotic seduction. She it is who with her sweet barb arouses the love of Medea (Pindar, *Pyth.*, IV, 219) and who possesses the secret keys of divine love (*Pyth.*, IX, 39). Nothing can resist the enchantment of divine Persuasion.

Soon, however, and without losing her Olympian guardianship of amorous seduction, *Peithô* is to prove to be the goddess of the persuasive efficacy of the word. Alcman (frag. 44 Diehl) declares her to be the daughter of Promethea, the sister of Tyche and Eunomia, and goddess of political persuasion. Her figure is now well defined by the opposition between her, *Peithô*, and *Bia* (Force) or *Anankê* (Necessity). Taking up that ancient tradition Herodotus, too, contrasts *Peithô* and *Anankaie* (VIII, 111); and a gloss to the *Orestes* of Euripides (1239) very significantly converts the daughter of Oceanus into the wife of Phoroneus, the founder of political and civil order. During the fifth century this very broad persuasive function of *Peithô* constantly became more and more evident. In the *Suppliants* Aeschylus presents to us the King of Argos commending himself to the protection of Persuasion and Fortune (sisters to one another, according to Alcman) in order to convince the assembly of his people with his words (*Suppl.*, 523); in the *Eumenides* the "venerable Peithô" lends sweetness and charm to the suasive speech of Athena (885), and under her enchanting gaze (Ibycus, frag. 8: Peithô is *aganoblepharos*, "of gentle gaze") the tongue and the mouth of Orestes' divine mediatrix are triumphant. "Zeus Agoraios has won," Athena proclaims at the end of her able allegation (970–73). "Zeus Agoraios": the Zeus of public assemblies, the supreme god of the efficacious word. And under sophistic influence the Hecuba of Euripides will say: "To what end, mortals, the striving for knowledge and the investigation of it? Persuasion [*Peithô*] alone is sovereign over men. Why do we not work rather to acquire as wages the perfect science?" (*Hec.*, 816). More than the marble buildings in which the gods are worshipped, the word is the true temple of Peithô, Euripides concludes (*Antigone*, frag. 170 N). For a Greek nothing could express more forcefully and effectively the connection between persuasion and the word.

But the influence of the goddess is not always beneficent, because the seduction of the human word can also be corrupting. By undoing the old antithesis between *Bia* and *Peithô* Aeschylus will say that at times "deadly persuasion" overpowers (*biatai*) man (*Agam.*, 385) and will call the divine daughter of Oceanus "deceptive" (*Coeph.*, 726). The work of *Peithô* has the same pejorative sense in Sophocles (*El.*, 562; *Trach.*, 661, frag. 781–86). It is possible that, as Peek notes,[42] this negative regard for verbal persuasion may not be unrelated to the political fate of Athens so often led astray by oratory during the fifth century. The fact is that Aristophanes' comic view of the goddess of persuasion belongs to the declining years of this century. Persuasion serves to give an appearance of justice to what is said, cunningly points out the Coryphaeus of the *Clouds* (1938). Nothing, however, is so revealing of the new popular feeling as a poetic contest in the *Frogs* between Eurip-

---

[42] W. Peek, "Peitho," R.E. *19*, 1, col. 204. I refer the reader to this excellent article for bibliography and epigraphic and archeological sources in respect to the goddess *Peithô*.

ides and Aeschylus in the presence of Dionysus. "Persuasion has no other temple than the word," says Euripides, quoting the famous verse in his *Antigone*. Aeschylus replies in a verse of his *Niobe:* "Of the gods, only Thanatos does not love those present" (frag. 156). Which of those two verses can be the weightier? Dionysus solves the question by speaking thus: "Persuasion is a giddy thing and has no brains [*noun ouk echon*]" (*Frogs,* 1391–96). It can well be observed that the Sophists and Socrates—the *Frogs* was performed in the year 405—have visited Athens: the art of convincing by the word has not given the Athenians all that they expected of it.

Peithô, goddess of amorous seduction and persuasive speech, the "august" *Peithô* (Hesiod), "sweet-eyes" (Ibycus), "wise" (Pindar), "enchanting," "venerable" (Aeschylus), and "sovereign" (Euripides), was nothing but a personification of the psychological and social efficacy of the word. "The power of argument," *die Macht der Gründe*, Wilamowitz calls *Peithô*, forgetting perhaps that the strength of human speech is not only logical and polemic.[43] The great importance that speaking well had for the Greek people since the time of their appearance on the historical scene is sanctified and deified in the form of this goddess Persuasion.[44] For the man of Greece there was something divine in the feat of convincing and shining socially by means of the word; and once the rationalizing and secularizing spirit of the fifth century has reduced what once had been "divine" to being merely "important"—all of that which is important to men began by being divine in a previous period of history—the great frequency of the terms *peithô*, "persuasion," and *peithein*, "to persuade," in literary texts will disclose unequivocally the old sacral, and in a way erotic, regard for the power of the word.[45] The pleasure of persuading

43. *Der Glaube der Hellenen*, 1, 32.
44. That personification must have taken place in post-Homeric Greece. Recall what was said of the silence of the epic with respect to *Peithô*.
45. The work of Euripides, in which these terms appear no less than one hundred seventy-two times (I owe this information to the careful compilation of J. T. Allen and G. Italie in *A Concordance to Euripides*, Berkeley and Los Angeles, 1954), proves it quite clearly. Let this example suffice.

by speaking must have been in the soul of the ancient Greeks an emotion religiously and psychologically connected with sexual pleasure. *Eros* and *logos* acquired a significant unity in the figure of the goddess *Peithô*.[46] But soon the divine becomes human: the idea of rhetoric that Corax and Gorgias are to propose to the Greeks—rhetoric as a "demiurge of persuasion"— will be but the result to which the secularization of that ancient Oceanid divinity necessarily had to lead.

The word of man is divine and pleasurable not only because it expresses and communicates, but also because it persuades. The persuasive word is pacifying (Aeschylus, *Persians*, 837), gentle (Sophocles, *Philoct.*, 629), beautiful (*Philoct.*, 1268), enchanting (Euripides, *Andr.*, 290), and only very firm and keen minds can resist the power of its enchantment (Aeschylus, *Seven*, 715). What then is the human word? What does the word mean in the life of man? How does it act upon the one who utters it and the one who hears it? What are the limits of its action? The Sophists, and later Socrates, Plato, and Aristotle, will meditate persistently and profoundly upon these themes. But the thought of the Sophists and the philosophers had as its instigation and its basic assumption that very lofty Greek regard for speech of which the lyric poets and tragedians give us such clear evidence. It would be foolish to expect from those poets a systematic doctrine regarding the psychological and social action of the word, but it is not impossible nor does it seem inopportune to collect in orderly fashion some of the ideas described by them in regard to that action —ideas that doubtless circulated through the minds of Athens during the middle decades of the fifth century.

I shall limit myself to the tragic authors. The "word" expresses the being and the innermost nature of man (Sophocles, *Oed. Col.*, 1188) and makes one who rightly uses it a "seer" (*Oed. Col.*, 74). But when it acts as a means of communication among men, what function does it perform? Two

---

46. Rendered roughly and unilaterally libidinous, the same intuition lies at the root of the psychoanalytical reduction of the pleasure of speaking—and even of the function of speech—to a type of oral eroticism.

principal and mutually opposed resources may give concrete reality and order to human social existence: force and the word. The serious and permanent social problem of the opposition, or the complementary nature, of word and force deeply preoccupies Sophocles. "Who commands here by word and by force?" asks Oedipus upon arriving in Colonus (*Oed. Col.*, 68). Force, in the sense of compulsion, and word, or persuasion, are a constant conceptual pair in the plot of *Philoctetes* (563, 593–94, 612); and when Polynices in *Oedipus at Colonus* describes his banishment by Eteocles he will have recourse to those two terms to show his brother's injustice: "Eteocles has expelled me from the land without having overcome me by the word [he means: by his eloquence] and without having vied with me with his hands and with his works" (1295–98). Force and speech mutually oppose and complement one another. But is one of the two terms superior to the other? A speech of Ulysses in *Philoctetes* gives the reply of Sophocles and perhaps of the entire Greek people: "In the life of men it is the tongue [that is, the word] and not the act, that governs all" (98–99). *Peithô* must prevail over *Bia*.[47]

Words, vigorous and persuasive words: they are the key to interhuman relations and success in the city. A word can have the power of an arrow (Aeschylus, *Coeph.*, 380–81) and penetrate into the inner depths of the heart of one who hears it (*Coeph.*, 451–53). The prudent man should seek his good renown by means of the word, without forgetting that excessively beautiful speeches—relying, accordingly, more upon the beauty of their form than the efficacy of their persuasion—often destroy cities (Euripides, *Hippol.*, 486–89) and that good conduct is the best resource for speaking well (*Hec.*, 1238–39). An artful speech is the worst of plagues (Aeschylus, *Prom.*, 685–86); well-composed speeches, on the other hand, whether they enchant, or anger, or move to pity, lend voice to the

47. Later, and as a result of philosophy, *Peithô* will even come to assume the role of *Bia* and *Anankê*, because the truth necessarily forces us to accept her when the *logos*, the word, acquaints us with her. Hence Plato will be able to speak of a "necessary" or "irresistible persuasion," *peithô anankaia* (*Soph.*, 265d).

silent man (Sophocles, *Oed., Col.*, 1281–83), especially if the one who utters them is a man of prestige: "Speech," Euripides will teach, "does not have the same power in the mouth of obscure men as in that of renowned men" (*Hec.*, 293–95). A friend's word warms the heart (*Med.*, 143). Finally, the sorrowing man gains some consolation by voicing his sorrow in the presence of another (*Philoct.*, 692–94).

Can it then be surprising that the word, an instrument so powerful in modifying and governing man's reality, should by itself, without the addition of a magical power, have the ability to achieve the cure of human disease or at least to help in it? Faintly presaged in the "cheering speech" of the cures of Nestor and Patroclus, the therapy of the word—no longer a magic therapy, but natural—continues to be mentioned in the literature of the fifth century. Oceanus says to Prometheus, in Aeschylus' tragedy: "Do you not know, Prometheus, that there are speeches that cure [*iatroi logoi*] the sickness of wrath?" To which the Enchained One replies: "Yes, if one knows how to pacify the heart at the right times instead of persisting in drying up by force [*bia*] a spirit full of wrathful humor" (*Prom.*, 377–80). From our point of view, that passage—to the internal dialectic of which the now well-known opposition between the word and force belongs—is of inestimable value: an especially violent disorder of the passions now receives the name of a "sickness," and is conceived of as an affection both psychic and somatic of human reality, in accordance with the sense of the term *thymos* in the anthropology of ancient Greece,[48] and perhaps by comparing the action of the word to that of a soothing and attenuating massage, its therapeutic power over the morbid "swelling" of the spirit brought on by the wrathful humor, *sphringônta thymon*, is openly stated. The timely word of the physician, and, in general, of a friend, can be a *iatros logos*, and not only because it sometimes cures or relieves but also because it teaches and consoles. "It is

48. Beside the books of Snell and Onians already cited, see *Le vocabulaire médical d'Eschyle et les écrits hippocratiques*, by J. Dumortier (Paris, 1935).

sweet for the ill to know clearly what they yet have to suffer," says Aeschylus (*Prom.*, 698–99) with deep insight. From a strictly medical point of view this thought of Aeschylus completes his famous *pathei mathos:* the maxim according to which one learns only through pain. Now we are told that the pain of the patient can be "sweet"—within the limits of the sweetness which the pain allows, of course—if it comes to be "known," if the sufferer succeeds in "giving it its proper place" in his own life through the words of one who understands his pain and his illness better than he.

Euripides too knows that the word can cure. A victim of her sick passion, Phaedra exclaims: "Oh deadly and wretched fate of womankind! What arts, what words have we to loose the embrace of the misfortune which has overthrown us?" (*Hippol.*, 668–71). But this social inferiority of women in regard to the "arts" and the "words" which aid to beguile misfortunes would be psychologically compensated by the greater adaptability of the feminine character to the healing, "enchanting," action of the timely word. In the tragedy named for her, Andromache gives her reply to the Phaedra of *Hippolytus:* "It is in the nature of women to enchant [*terpsis*] present ills by keeping them ever on their tongue and lips" (*Andr.*, 93–95). Hector's wife is referring, as is obvious from the context, to the psychological workings of the spoken complaint; but it is plain that her thought has as its corollary the curative or consoling action of the heard word. The word able to aid "from the mouth," insofar as it is uttered, aids also "from the ear," insofar as it is merely heard.

But the tragic poets are not unaware of the relative narrowness of the limitation which Nature has placed upon the psychological and curative efficacy of the word. Aeschylus asserts through the mouth of the King of Argos (*Suppl.*, 514) that when fear is too great, there are no words that can overcome it, and Sophocles' Electra knows, for her part, that for her there can be no word of avail (*El.*, 225–28). The reality of man is frequently more powerful than the human word, even though the strength of the latter may be so great on occasion.

Peithô, Persuasion, is often overcome by *Bia*, Violence, or by *Ananké*, Necessity. Back in the excited and confused years of the sixth century the sagacious Theognis had already said: "If the sons of Asclepius had received from the gods the power to cure the evil and perversity of men, what rich profits they would gain! If good sense were something that could be produced or instilled into man, the son of an honorable father, whom wise speeches had persuaded, would never become a villain" (I, 430-36).

In relation to our problem—the possible psychological and curative efficacy of the human word—a swarm of grave questions besieges the minds of Athens in the second half of the fifth century. Are the perversity and disorder of the passions "diseases" of man in the strict sense of the term? And if they are, to what extent do they belong to his nature, to his *physis*? Against *physis* in general and against the *physis* of man in particular, what can the *logos* accomplish, in its twofold dimension of reason and word? And how can that action of the *logos* be transformed into *techné*, into "art" or "technique"? In the life of man where does that which is nature, *physis*, end and where does that which is convention or law, *nomos*, begin? Philosophers, Sophists, and physicians will strive to give a satisfactory reply to this difficult list of questions.

III. Wisdom or Sophia, Xavier Zubiri has written, adopted two forms in the Greece of the fifth century: The one form pathetic: tragedy; the other neotic: philosophy.[49] Both being deeply rooted in the same historic soil, the ancient Greek mentality, the former was the work of the continental Greeks and the latter a creation of the colonial Greeks. Attica and Ionia, each in its own way, were the cradle of Hellenic classicism; I mean to say, of that which is classic for us in ancient Greece.

Howald[50] has contrasted the deep religiosity of the continental Greeks and the scanty religiosity of the colonial Greeks. The religious movements of the eighth and seventh centuries,

---

49. *Naturaleza, Historia, Dios* (Madrid, 1944), p. 226.
50. "Kultur der Antike," *Handbuch der Kulturgeschichte*, ed. by Kindermann (Potsdam, 1936).

which so profoundly stir the Hellenic world—the cult of Dionysus, Orphism, the mysteries—hardly reach Ionia, or reach it in a very weakened form. Archilochus, the poet of Paros, wishes to sing a dithyramb while drunk, which is blasphemy, for the dithyramb should be sung by a chorus. Pythagoras founds his Orphic sect in Magna Graecia; in Samos, his homeland, he would not have found a favorable soil. Xenophanes, on the other hand, knew well how to express the rational attitude of his Ionic world toward traditional religion. Thus, the inner insecurity and the deep sense of guilt of the ancient Greeks are not expressed religiously among the Ionians, as in peninsular Greece, but in the longing for awareness of participating in a cosmic harmony humanly knowable and known. "The idea and the desire to find in the cosmos the harmony that he lacked in his inner world," Howald concludes, "led Thales of Miletus and his successors, the so-called pre-Socratic philosophers, to concern themselves with nature beyond practical needs. Such was the Ionic form of religious experience . . . But the harmony thus postulated should not depend upon a belief but must be demonstrated by experiment and logical conclusion; it should be accessible to reason, it should be *true*. In this way the concept of truth came into the world—with the cosmic symbol, which lasted but a short while."

Accurate as a whole, Howald's account must be refined. Philosophy was not an expression of *irreligiousness* or the intellectual face of a collective *asebeia;* as compared to peninsular Greece the thought of the Ionians was rather a consequence of *another religiosity*. Theognis too, a nobleman of Megara, knows how to confront Zeus boldly and doubt his justice at the height of the sixth century. The Greek emigrant took with him his ancient gods and his traditional worship to the coast of Asia Minor, and there is more than one reason to suppose that Apollo in Miletus, Artemis in Ephesus, and Hera in Samos were as venerated as in their temples of Attica, Boeotia, and Thessaly. But the truth is that the psychological and social conditions of colonial life—a colony is, above all, a group of men both obliged and resolved to live by themselves—came to create in the Greek mind a type of religiosity and intellectual daring which, on one hand traditional, on the other implied a considerable novelty, and led in the end to the idea of divinity dominant among the pre-Socratic *physiologoi*. Not in vain could Thales of Miletus say, according to Aristotle (*de anima*, 411 a 7), that "everything is full of gods," and it was not by chance that Werner Jaeger could write a book accurately titled, *The Theology of the First Greek Philosophers*. More than the intellectual aspect of habitual and collective *asebeia*, Ionic philosophy was the theoretical form of a new type of *eusebeia*, that one in whose virtue Hippocrates could deem himself more "pious" than the superstitious quacks given to the practice of charms and purifications.[51]

Something similar must be said of the conception of Greek history underlying an expression that W. Nestle has made famous: *Vom Mythos zum Logos*.[52] Greek classicism may be the work of a transition from the "mythical" to the "logical," from one way of living in which the word of man names images to another in which it expresses concepts. In general terms this is true; but it is also true, and Nestle himself readily recognizes it, that Greek thought never could nor would dispense with the myth. It is not even necessary to resort to the example of Plato, the great poet of myth. Did not Aristotle himself, so ascetically conceptual in his philosophy, once confess that solitude and isolation were making him an ever greater friend of myths? (frag. 668 Rose). It would be more accurate to say that Ionic thought was the transition from a preponderantly mythical *logos* to a preponderantly noetic *logos;* a transition in which the Greeks came to discover that if human knowledge

---

51. Howald, for example, places in contrast the "belief" of the peninsular Greeks and the "experimental and reasoning attitude" of the colonial Greeks. But was there not perhaps in the latter a new form of the Greek manner of believing? Did not Parmenides perhaps, who can serve as one example, speak of a *pistis alêthês* (true belief) and of *pistios ischys* (the power of belief)? (Diels, B 1, 30 and B 8, 12).

52. I allude to the author's excellent book of this title (Stuttgart, 1940).

begins with the myth it is obliged to end in it, if it would be wholly faithful to the impulse which quickens it from within.

I need not expound here the genesis of Ionic philosophy: that poorly known process by virtue of which some men of Miletus passed from *mythologia* to *physiologia* in the middle decades of the sixth century.[53] Faithful to the circumscribed area of my subject, I shall limit myself to showing how the pre-Socratic philosophers thought of and understood the psychological and curative action of the human word. To this end, as in the previous section, I shall study successively the magical and the natural utilization of the word, the charm, and persuasive speech.

The inquiry has to begin with Pythagoras and his school. Who was Pythagoras and what was he? Plunging boldly into the ethnological and historico-religious background of the *vita pythagorica*, today there are not a few who answer this question by saying: Pythagoras was primarily a Greek shaman. The contact of the Greek world with Thrace and its colonial opening upon the Black Sea must have brought shamanism into the body of the rising Greek culture. Rohde's famous phrase about Orphism and the cult of Dionysus—"a drop of alien blood in the veins of the Greeks"—must extend to other forms of religiosity and not be restricted geographically by the parochial notion of invariably attributing to the Orient and to the South the source of that which in Hellenic culture does not appear to be wholly Greek.[54] A whole series of figures in ancient Greece, some more legendary, others more historic—Abaris of Hyperboreus, Aristeas of Proconnesus, Hermotimus of Clazomenae, Epimenides, Zamolxis, and perhaps Orpheus himself—must have been the result of that early shamanistic

---

53. I refer the reader to explanations by Burnet, Cornford, Zubiri, Jaeger, Gigon, Nestle, etc., and of course to the texts of the pre-Socratic thinkers themselves. I shall always quote them from the fifth edition, prepared by W. Kranz, of the *Fragmente der Vorsokratiker* of H. Diels (Berlin, 1934).

54. See the aforementioned works of Meuli, Dodds, Boyancé, Nilsson, and Eliade.

"vaccination" of the old Hellenes. Recall what has been said on previous pages in regard to the *iatromantes*.

What is a shaman? Within a historico-religious morphology constructed with precision and rigor a shaman is a man who, after having felt within himself a religious call and after having undergone a period of "professional" apprenticeship, comes to possess technical ability for a number of activities: falling into an ecstatic trance, magic flight (ascents, descents, and voyages of the soul during that trance), dominion over spirits and dominion over fire (M. Eliade). The shaman, accordingly, is at once a seer, charmer, medicaster, and master of life. His function in primitive societies would have allowed him to be called truly "an expert in remedying the precariousness and impurity of human existence."

It would be useless to seek in ancient Greece "morphologically pure" shamans such as those who up to a few years ago practiced among the Tongus, Yakuts, Buriats, and Samoyeds of Siberia. But it is not hard to find shaman-like traits mixed in at times with "oriental" elements in a goodly number of Greek figures, institutions, and legends, beginning with those named and continuing with others, such as that concerning the Centaurs.[55] Such is the case with the figure of Pythagoras. We know very little with certainty about the life and the doctrine of this man. But a thoughtful examination of the luxuriant "Pythagorean legend" has made it possible to discover or at least to suppose on a very firm basis that the sage of Samos belongs to the realm of shamanism. Several motifs of this legend—previous incarnations of the soul of Pythagoras (Heraclides Ponticus, cited by Diogenes Laertius), descent to Hades, ascent to a cloud (Ovid), relations with Zamolxis (Herodotus),[56] power over *daimônes* (Iamblicus)—give considerable likelihood to

55. In the excellent book *Le problème des Centaures*, by G. Dumézil (Paris, 1929) initiations of a shamanistic character are described. The memory of the medical wisdom of the Centaur Chiron comes at once to mind.

56. M. Eliade does not accept the shamanistic status of Zamolxis, though he does in the case of Pythagoras (pp. 351–53).

the supposition of a shamanistic initiation of the "philosopher" of Samos. In it Pythagorean medicine must have had one of its main roots.[57]

Whatever may have been the relation of Pythagoreanism to the Orphic movement,[58] the similarity between the magical medicine of the Pythagoreans and the "cures" effected by the followers of Orpheus is unquestionable. Three features, in fact, appear to characterize the therapeutic procedure of Pythagoras and his disciples: the intention of expelling *daimônes* from the body and soul of the patient, the use of music, and the cathartic conception of diet. Let us now turn our attention to the first two.

The most ancient Pythagorean ideas regarding disease were crudely primitive: according to them, a victim of illness must be a man possessed and defiled by some malign *daimôn* (Diog. Laer., VIII, 32).[59] In consequence, the intention of the medical treatment must be primarily apotropaic (expulsion of the disturbing *daimôn*) and cathartic (restoration of the na-

---

57. On the "problem of Pythagoras" the publications of A. Delatte, *Études sur la littérature pythagoricienne* (Paris, 1915), *Essai sur la politique pythagoricienne* (Liège, 1922), and *La Légende de Pythagore de Diogène Laërce* (Bruxelles, 1922) should be read in particular. Also *La Légende de Pythagore: de Grèce en Palestine* (Paris, 1927), by I. Lévy, and *Quaestiones Pythagoreae, Orphicae, Empedocleae*, by Gu. Rathmann (Halle, 1933), and *Pythagoras und Orpheus*, by H. Kerény (Berlin, 1938). The bibliography in respect to the Pythagorean "philosophy" has been amply reviewed in Ueberweg's *Geschichte der Philosophie*, in Ferrater Mora's *Diccionario de Filosofía*, and in other similar publications.

58. This relation between Pythagoreanism and Orphism is commonly accepted. Rohde, Cornford, Nilsson, and Kerény assert it without reservation, and Guthrie does so somewhat more circumspectly. Delatte and Boyancé are less explicit. Without denying the value of the warnings which require a detailed examination of sources, to the lay reader the existence of a historical relationship between Pythagoras and Orpheus seems more than probable. The sociological considerations of Kerény in respect to such a relationship are very thought-provoking.

59. For the "demonic" interpretation of disease in ancient Greece see J. Tamborino, *De antiquorum daemonismo*, in R.G.V.V., 7, 3 (Giessen, 1909), and Ch. Michel "Les bons et les mauvais esprits dans les croyances populaires de la Grèce ancienne," in *Rev. d'hist. et litt. religeuses*, N.S. *1*, p. 291.

ture of the patient to its initial "purity"). A. Delatte has brought to light the great similarity between the superstitious therapy of the charlatans and quacks combatted in the work *de morbo sacro* and the medicinal and ritual practices of the Pythagoreans. "The remedies of those charlatans," Boyancé comments, "are aimed at a particular ailment but in themselves are practices of very general application; all occurs as if the *Pythagorean life* were being propounded by them as necessary to avoid epilepsy." A twofold conjecture, in the form of a dilemma, arises in the mind of the historian: either the cathartists mentioned in Hippocrates' work are unworthy heirs of Pythagoras, or the Pythagoreans had accepted into their rule of life the beliefs and the rites which Hippocrates cites. Present knowledge does not permit us to choose with certainty between the two conjectures.[60]

In any case epilepsy and madness were not the only diseases attributed to the invasion of an unnamed or name-possessing *daimôn* into the body of the patient; the same was held of many other ailments, especially sudden and febrile ones,[61] including psychic affections of a nonmorbid type such as dreams and passions. For the primitive mind everything in the life of man that "happens" in an unexpected and incomprehensible way has as its hidden cause the penetration of a disturbing and invisible *daimôn* into his reality. Aristides Quintilian will say that certain "wise men"—it is more than probable that he is alluding to the Pythagoreans—call the passions "small epilepsies," [62] an expression which reveals very clearly the interpretation of intense emotional states as "small possessions," [63] and the unbroken transition that always ex-

60. Boyancé, pp. 106–07.
61. See in this respect, besides the monographs of Tamborino and Michel mentioned above, the work of A. Höfler in *Zentralblatt für Anthropologie, 1* (1900), 1.
62. *De musica*, III, XXV, p. 93, Jahn.
63. Just as the sneeze, a sudden loss of the "breath of life," is for the people of Andalusia a "tiny death." Ulysses (*Od.*, V, 468) must have thought likewise. In another sense Democritus calls the sexual act a "small apoplexy" (frag. 32 Diels, quoting Stobaeus) or a "small epilepsy" (Delatte).

isted for the Greek between *pathos* as "passion" and *pathos* as "illness." It will probably not be out of place to note that that transition had at the same time a quantitative character—for a very intense passion is already a morbid affection—and a genetic character—for diseases in the strict sense of the term produce passions, and passions can produce diseases or express themselves by the same symptoms as the latter.

Disease and the passions being so conceived, what might be their treatment? The primitive Pythagoreans, like so many other "primitives", appealed to the presumed magic efficacy of the charm and of music, more precisely, to the sung charm. Aristoxenus of Tarentum said that the Pythagoreans purified the body with medicine and the soul with music (*Anecd. Paris.*, Cramer, *1*, 172). But it is certain that this precise cathartic and therapeutic dichotomy comes from the methodical mentality of Aristoxenus, for both Iamblichus (*Vita Pythag.*, 164) as well as Porphyry (*Vita Pythag.*, 33 and 64) tell us very clearly that diseases of the body also were treated by the Pythagoreans by means of music. The music of the lyre—Pythagoras rejected the flute, as Plato did later: the blowing of this instrument "would defile" the ear of those who listen to it—was the main device of the magical medicine of Pythagoras and his followers. In the Pythagorean school there was even a sort of musical pharmacopoeia, an art of mixing sounds wholly comparable to that of mixing simple medicaments aimed, like the latter, at achieving special therapeutic effects. The analogy between this practice and the one which Hoffman was able to observe among the Ojibway Indians is noteworthy: "In the course of the preparatory instruction making up the first stage of the initiation the teacher teaches the pupil particularly effective songs, but he learns also to 'prepare' songs for the needs of his practice, exactly as a student of pharmacy would learn to compound medicaments."[64]

Does this mean that the human word played no role at all in the musical enchantments of the Pythagoreans? The truth is that such enchantments, like those of the Orpheans, were al-

64. Cited by J. Combarieu, *La musique et la magie*, p. 78.

most always songs and that in them the words were no less important than the music. Iamblichus and Porphyry speak textually of *epôdai* when they explain the therapeutic activities of Pythagoras. Accompanying himself on the lyre, the Pythagorean magician sought the expulsion of the *daimôn* and the purificatory cure of the patient by singing paeans of Thaletas and passages from Homer and Hesiod, more or less close in content to the case treated. Iamblichus relates, for example, that a drunk and violently enamored young man was brought to a paroxysm of his double passion by the performance of a flute player who was playing his instrument in the Phrygian mode. Pythagoras, having been called to aid the youth, cured him by substituting for the sound of the flute the grave strain of a spondaic measure (*Vita Pythag.*, 112). The sacral and theological character which the poetry of Homer and Hesiod had for the men of Greece—"the Bible of the Greeks," Wilamowitz has called that poetry—well explains the preference of those who sought in it the text of their charms. Centuries later Proclus will inherit that old Pythagorean practice and will even use it on his own person. One day on which a violent pain was tormenting him he had certain hymns sung and his pains were allayed.[65] The morning and evening purifications of the followers of Pythagoras had, to all appearances, the same antidemonic purpose. In the morning those purifications eliminated from the soul the confusion created by nocturnal *daimônes* and the bad dreams which the latter might have been able to cause; in the evening they prepared the way for the good *daimônes*, the good dreams, and blocked the access of the evil ones.[66]

It seems reasonable, according to this, to attribute some shamanistic traits to Pythagoras. In a certain measure the founder of Pythagoreanism was a kinsman of Abaris, Aristeas, and Hermotimus of Clazomenae. But the figure of Pythagoras would

65. Marinus, *Vita Procli.*, 20, p. 161, 21 Boissonade.
66. To the aforecited bibliography should be added the dissertation of S. N. Newhall *Quid de somnis censuerunt quoque modo eis usi sint quaeritur* (Harvard, 1923).

remain lamentably misunderstood and degraded should it be forgotten that if in a way he was a shaman, he was one without at all losing his quality as a Greek. He made magic use of music but he did so—no other man had gone so far before him —by orienting his mind toward what music "is"; if he conceived of the passions of the soul and the fact of disease in a primitive and demonic manner, his intelligence, brilliantly heedful of a rigorous understanding of what things "are," came for the first time to formulate, or at least to prepare, a truly "scientific" doctrine regarding disease.[67] Without ceasing to be a magician and a sorcerer in the broadest sense of these words, Pythagoras is a historic landmark decisive in the process leading from magic medicine to scientific medicine.

What is music? In its own essence, independently of the effects that hearing it produces in us, music is at once *sound* and *number,* for the pitch of the sound of a musical string is in strict numerical relationship to its length. A feat of Pythagoras' genius: with this discovery of his the magical action of music is brought into direct relation with the magical action of number.[68] But this is not all. Music is harmonious when it imitates the harmony of the movement of the stars; and since the stars are the most divine part of divine Nature, it follows therefore that number must possess a significance and a value at once religious and cosmic. "For the Pythagoreans," Aristotle will later say, "numbers are the essence of all things, and the heavens harmony and number" (*Met.*, A, 5, 985b 23). Number must be the principle and the foundation of the cosmos.

Accordingly, the good health of man, in its twofold psychic and somatic sense, is divine purity and harmony. "So that his soul might always be imbued with divinity Pythagoras

67. The consideration of things from the point of view of their "being" does not begin in an "explicit" way, as Zubiri has made clear, until Parmenides and Heraclitus ("Sócrates y la sabiduría griega," in *Naturaleza, Historia, Dios*), but "implicitly" it was already in the speculations of the Greek thinkers prior to them.

68. The problem of the relations between the "metaphysics of number" of the Pythagoreans and the wisdom of Persia will not be discussed. I limit myself to referring the reader to the works of Reitzenstein, Götze, and Kranz.

... was accustomed to sing with the cithara" (Censorinus, *de die natali*, 3). This statement by Censorinus well expresses the true sense of the Pythagorean songs—simultaneously magical, moral, metaphysical, and religious—and enables us to understand in considerable depth the ideas concerning the passions and illness germinating in Magna Graecia toward the end of the fifth century.

Disease, violent emotional states, and dreams are "passions" (*pathê*) of man produced by *daimónes* invading the individual reality of the one who undergoes them. Such appears to be the *cause* of these disturbances. But what can their real substance be? What do the disturbances of human life which we call passion and disease *consist* of? The reply of the Pythagoreans is foreseeable. Violent passions and diseases, they will tell us, are "lacks of harmony," disorders of the number to which the divine purity of man ultimately can and must be reduced, the conformity of his life to the universal order of Nature and good health. The *vita pythagorica*—diet, songs, science of number, various precepts—would be the method to preserve the divine harmony of health or to win it back if by chance a violent *pathos* has caused us to lose it. One can already sense the imminence of the "physiological pathology" of Alcmeon of Crotona, with its fertile idea of *isonomia* (equal distribution, balance).[69]

Let us now return to the text of Iamblichus: "The Pythagoreans used more salves and poultices than their predecessors; they did not set much store by treatment with drugs; they almost always used the former only on ulcers; even less did they resort to incisions and cautery; in some diseases they also used magical songs [sung charms, *epôdai*]" (*Vita Pythag.*, 163-64). In those songs, what role did the words of the singer play, together with the music? How did Pythagoras interpret the magical workings of the sung word? How could that which might be said in the song contribute to the reestablishment of lost harmony? The truth is that the mind of Pythagoras, still too ar-

69. For Pythagorean medicine see particularly the chapter on Pythagoras in *Antike Medizin*, by J. Schumacher (Berlin, 1940).

chaic, had neither reached the point at which it could ask itself these questions nor was it capable of giving them an adequate reply. To obtain this, it will be necessary to wait for Plato.

The use of the magic word in the therapy of Empedocles was as unquestionable as in the medical treatments of Pythagoras. He himself states so clearly in his *Katharmoi* or Doctrine of purification: "Men follow me by thousands to find out whither the benefit of the path [the way of salvation] leads, some in need of oracles; others, because of the most varied diseases, wish to hear a curative word, long tormented by great pains" (frag. 112 Diels). Uttered by Empedocles and recalled by him with boastful praise in the *Katharmoi*, what other than a magic charm could that "curative word" (*euêkês baxis*) of which we are told here have been? Does not a man who at that moment feels himself very close to being an "incorruptable god" perchance proclaim it? Diogenes Laertius, supported by the testimony of Satyrus, states that Gorgias claimed to have been present when Empedocles was practicing sorcery (*goêteuonti*) (*Diog.*, VIII, 59). Even more explicit is Iamblichus' account. A certain young man wished to kill a guest of Empedocles by the name of Anchitos; Empedocles, accompanying himself on the lyre, sang the passage from the *Odyssey* which begins with the verse, "*Nepenthês* [the drug so called] against tears and wrath, which causes all woes to be forgotten" (*Od.*, IV, 220), and succeeded in dissuading the man who was plotting the murder from his intent (*Vita Pythag.*, 113). There can be no doubt that the "curative words" of which Empedocles—magician, physician, poet, philosopher, seer, and politician—tells us can only be *epôdai*, in the most direct and traditional sense of the term.

But, as in the case of Pythagoras and with even firmer basis, the magic logotherapy of Empedocles must be understood without losing view of the whole personality of the one who utilized it. The sage of Agrigentum was indeed a complex and singular figure, on the one hand a true shaman and the author of an ardent religious and purificatory poem, the "Purifications"; on the other, the keen-sighted naturalist and the profound philosopher of the poem, "On Nature." What should we think of him? Was Empedocles a shaman, a cathartist, and a magician who evolved subsequently toward natural science, as Bidez and Kranz assert, or was he a man of science later converted to Orphism and Pythagoreanism, as Diels and Wilamowitz suppose? Both hypotheses are possible. But it is also possible to imagine something more simple and likely, namely that in the person of Empedocles, as in that of Pythagoras, there were blended in vital and historic unity two mental attitudes only incompatible when we translate them into our present ways of thinking, so paradigmatic of the "rational" and the "irrational" and definitely so removed from those current in Sicily and in Magna Graecia during the first half of the fifth century.[70]

Empedocles sees in the cosmos a reality at once single and multiple, permanent and plastic.[71] Pythagoras, Orphism, Parmenides, and Heraclitus weigh heavily upon his mind. The

70. This is the authoritative opinion of Ettore Bignone in his *Empedocle* (Turin, 1916). "The complexity of the inner world of Empedocles", W. Jaeger writes on his part, "is evidently something more than a purely individual question: it reflects in an especially impressive way the many internal strata of the culture of Sicily and Magna Graecia . . . The fact that such diverse intellectual elements were already traditionally on hand and ready to be welded together within the same individual could not fail to give rise to a new type, a synthesizer, with a philosophical personality. It is not surprising therefore that the spirit of Empedocles is of extraordinary breadth and inner tension" (*La teología de los primeros filósofos griegos*, p. 133).

71. An explanation of the cosmology and the physiology of Empedocles would be out of place here; consult the histories of Greek philosophy (Zeller, Ueberweg, Burnet, etc.). The figure and the work of Empedocles have been recently studied, not including the above-mentioned works of Bignone and Jaeger, by W. Kranz (*Empedokles*, Zürich, 1949), and J. Zafiropulo (*Empédocle d'Agrigente*, Paris, 1953). A. Delatte has devoted some pages to the Empedoclean idea of frenzy in his monograph *Les conceptions de l'enthousiasme chez les philosophes présocratiques* (Paris, 1934). In one of his final works—that titled, "Terminating and Interminable Analysis"—Freud makes of Empedocles his predecessor: the two powers Love and Discord, which according to Empedocles rule the cosmos, were probably equivalent to the two protoinstincts of Freudian analysis, Eros and Destruction. See the profound and thought-provoking work of J. Rof Carballo "Freud y Empédocles de Agrigento," *Revista de Psiquiatría y Psicología médica de Europa y América latinas*, 2 (1956), 725–45.

fourfold multiplicity of the elements or "roots" of things, and the plasticity which the interplay of the two powers—*Philotês* and *Neikos*, Love and Discord—that rule over it gives to their movements, are ultimately ordained in the supreme, divine, unique, and quiescent harmony of the *Sphairos*, the latter a clear reminiscence of the "sphere" of Parmenides. But this is not the decisive part; from our present point of view the decisive part is that the man Empedocles feels himself personally and dramatically included in the process of the cosmos. "I have been a young man and a girl and a shrub and a bird and a mute fish that has leaped from the sea," one of his more famous statements says (frag. 117). The man who says this is not a humbug or a madman; he is a man who in the depth of his soul knows and feels his living community with the reality of the universe and with all the forms which the cyclical movement of that reality successively adopts. The cosmological knowledge of the philosopher and the purificatory doctrine of the "deified man," the *theios anêr*, are but two different modes of the same Sophia, the theoretical mode and the soteriological mode.

In both cases, in the *Peri physeôs* and in the *Katharmoi*, that Sophia is for Empedocles the result of a divine revelation by the Muse (frags. 3 and 131) and accordingly an object of belief, of faith (*pistis*). "I know that the truth dwells in these words which I am about to utter; but the truth is hard for men and only with labor does the offer of *belief* reach their soul" (frag. 114), state the "Purifications." In the case of this poem such a way of thinking and speaking does not surprise us. But is that expression not indeed repeated in the cosmological poem? The allusion to the "faith" with which its doctrine must be received is in it extremely obvious. "Do not believe your sight more than your hearing, nor place your murmuring ear above the subtle definitions of your tongue; and of the other organs, insofar as they lead to knowledge, do not deny belief to any" (frag. 3). The teachings of the Muse, of the Divinity, are *pistomata*, which we might call, as it were, "acts of faith," or "firm beliefs," knowledge which is the object of *pistis* (frag.

4); and when Empedocles utters to Pausanias, to whom the poem *Peri physeôs* is addressed, the supreme knowledge—or the supreme lack of knowledge—regarding the origin of things, he ends thus: "Know this clearly: you have heard the discourse of a god, *theou mython*" (frag. 23). For Empedocles, in short, to know is to believe and to believe is to know.

This is so because the knowledge that the sage of Agrigentum is expounding refers to the divine government and the divine essence of Nature, to which man as a being capable of deification belongs. Therefore the act of knowing and telling the truth has its seat and root in the depths of a pure heart (frag. 110). It is significant that Empedocles repeatedly uses the term *prapides*, "diaphragm"—or, if you will, "heart"— (frags. 110 and 129) for the "powers" or "faculties" both intellective and affective, which are put into intense play in the case of gifted acquisition of knowledge: body and soul are stirred and exalted when man comes to know, through labor and purity, the divine core of reality. Knowing thus, the *logos* is a sort of master key to the control of Nature. Solemnly does the final fragment of *Peri physeôs* proclaim this. Medicaments against illness and old age, mastery over the wind, drought, and rain, and even some power over death: all this will he attain who knows how to hear with faith the revealing and saving word of the sage.

Doubtlessly the talent of Empedocles for verbal seduction was very great. Diogenes Laertius declares him to have been the teacher of Gorgias, the creator of rhetoric. But in the eyes of the *iatromantes* of Agrigentum it is certain that that ability was merely an instrument and accoutrement. The important thing was the divine message to which his words gave expression. At the summit of humanity were to be found, together with princes, the *hymnopoloi* or composers of hymns, and the physicians (frag. 146). Now Empedocles was a seer, a composer of hymns, and a physician, that is, a man able to speak "with sanctified mouth" (frag. 3) and with it to utter words that save and heal those who know how to listen to them and make them theirs with understanding and faith. The ultimate sense of the *epôdai* of Empedocles must have been no other than this. In them magic was *also* religion and philosophy. But in this world subject to hatred, can a mortal man, even though his name be Empedocles of Agrigentum, succeed in making his word surely curative and redemptive? Shortly after the initial vaunt of the "Purifications"—"like an immortal god I walk among you"—the heartrending bitterness of the fourth fragment of that poem seems to give us a conclusive reply: "I too am now one of these, an exile from the gods and a wanderer —who has placed his trust in furious Discord" (frag. 115).

Pythagoras and Empedocles tried to cure the sick by magic charms. Heraclitus, on the other hand, seems to refer to these men with a touch of vituperation. One of his passages expresses thus the aristocratic feeling in his heart: "Then what are their mind and their understanding? The popular singers [*dêmôn aoidoisi*] fool them and they have the rabble for a master. They do not know this: that the many are bad and that only few are good" (frag. 104 Diels). What could those "popular singers" whom Heraclitus scorns have been but itinerant cathartists and reciters of *epôdai*, like the "charlatans and soothsayers" whom Plato will castigate in the *Republic*? Let us not believe, however, that the mind and the understanding of Heraclitus himself were totally free of archaic and, if you will, magic traits. For him disease had not ceased to be an impurity: "The souls of those who have fallen in war are purer than those of men who have died of disease" (frag. 136), he tells us through a commentator of Epictetus. A curative treatment would thus be to a certain extent the purification, *catharsis*, of the patient. There is still something of the Homeric Ulysses, of the Ulysses of Book I of the *Iliad*, in Heraclitus.[72] And, on the other hand, was not the sage of Ephesus a devout believer in the oracles of Delphi (frags. 92 and 93) to the point of asserting that in them the *Logos* of the universe became the *logos* of man, human reason, and word? [73]

[72]. The truth is that for the Greeks the treatment of disease was always "purification."
[73]. The attitude of Heraclitus toward "enthusiasm" and "frenzy" has been well studied by A. Delatte in *Les conceptions de l'enthousiasme*.

Among the Greek poets of the fifth century the words *epôdê* and *thelktêrion* began to be used in a metaphorical sense for the purpose of boldly and vigorously praising the great persuasive power of a speech or of any verbal expression. Recall what has been stated on previous pages. Accordingly, what occurred among the poets also takes place among the thinkers. But it does not seem an accident that it was the Sophists, and not the pre-Socratic philosophers, who were the first to make use of this significant stylistic innovation.

The *logos* of the philosophers, from Thales to Democritus, was used to declare what things "are." Moreover it should be stated, with Zubiri, that after Empedocles, Anaxagoras, and Democritus the *logos* means that which is understood and said rather than a mere saying or understanding, as it had up to then, and belongs therefore to the very structure of being. Empedocles will maintain for example that birds are, above all, fire. The "fire-thing" is on the one hand the *being* of the bird, but on the other hand it *gives us to understand* what the bird is; thus fire is at once the being of the bird and its reason, its *logos*. Things will be very different when the *logos*, as an instrument of human social intercourse, is principally used to convince or persuade others, or, as Zubiri says, when the "is" of conversation becomes the "is" of things.

> So long as man only looks at things and utters their names, he has nothing before his eyes but things. But as soon as he becomes a member of a dialogue, what things "are" shines through what the other man says. What I then have directly before my eyes are not the things, but the thoughts of the other man. The problems of being are changed automatically into problems of saying . . . And just as reasoning is what leads to the scientific *logos*, the *antilegein*, antilogy or controversy, leads directly to the technique of persuasion, which is something in the nature of the logic of opinion. Just as "to be" is "to appear", persuasion must "be" to cause one opinion to appear stronger than another. And this will be achieved when one suc-

ceeds in making the opponent waver, when one stirs his emotions. Reasoning will be replaced by discourse: it is Rhetoric.[74]

Since persuasion has come to have so much importance, it cannot be surprising that the persuasive power of the skillfully used word is now metaphorically called "charm," "incantation," and "witchery" (*epôdê, thelktêrion, goêteia*). Such was the case of Gorgias in his *Eulogy of Helen:* "Charms [*epoidai*] inspired by the word produce pleasure and banish pain; in fact, the power of the charm, intimately frequenting the fancy of the soul, seduces her [*ethelxe*], persuades her, transforms her by means of a sort of sorcery [*goêteiai*]" (*Enc. Hel.*, 10). Such too must have been the case of Thrasymachus, this "colossus of Chalcedon" who, according to the testimony of Plato, was able to enrage a throng and then calm it by the "charm" of his word (*Phaedrus*, 267c–d).

However this does not mean that it was the Sophists who revealed to the Greeks the social and moral importance of persuasion. The previous section has demonstrated this more than sufficiently. And like the lyric and tragic poets, the pre-Socratic thinkers and philosophers—Greeks, above all—were not remiss in rendering rational tribute to the holy prestige of the goddess *Peithô*.

The *logos*, in its double sense of word and reason, is the highest and the most specific of the gifts of human nature. By means of the *logos* man expresses what things are, shines in society, and is powerful in it by convincing others. Fair words and lofty deeds are the titles of social excellence in the Homeric epic. But as Heinimann has shown, in the fifth century the complementary relationship between word (*epos, mythos, logos, glotta*) and work (*ergon*) is served and there arises between these two concepts a relationship which is often antithetical. Word and work are not always joined to one another and on occasion oppose each other. "You harken to the speeches and the words of a clever man," Solon used to say to the Athenians, "and you do not regard any of the things [of the

74. *Naturaleza, Historia, Dios*, pp. 238 and 242.

"works": *ergón*] that happen" (frag. 8 Diehl, frag. 11 R. Adrados). Not a few Greek works of the fifth century will give literary expression to the same feeling. Spanish folk wisdom will later say that "Deeds and not fine words are proofs of love." [75]

Within the area circumscribed by the *logos-ergon* antithesis the different attitudes of the pre-Socratic thinkers and philosophers toward the problem of persuasion take shape. Even though at times the words of men deceive, the "human word" is not, for all that, a less admirable reality. Is not its very ability to lead men astray perhaps the best proof of its power? The *logos*, accordingly, will deserve all praise when, in the mouth of the philosopher, it expresses the truth of things and, in the mouth of the politician, makes violence useless and persuades men to act with justice. "Whatever you may have, have it by persuasion and not by force"; "Convince with good reason," the ancient maxim of Bias of Priene taught. In these maxims that opposition between "persuasion" and "force" to which I have referred in previous pages is evident. The rightly persuasive *logos* thus comes to occupy a "virtuous" mean between two extremes: on one hand, that against which the human word has no power, *Bia*, the blind and deaf violence of men, or *Ananké*, the invincible Necessity of natural movements; on the other hand, the deceptive *logos*, the deadly persuasion of words which entice into evil or error. Parmenides, for example, will once assert that "the way of persuasion follows the truth" (frag. 2 Diels) and again maintain that the language of men persuades them to admit things which do not correspond to true reality (frag. 8, 38–39). Parmenides could not be a total

75. F. Heinimann, *Nomos und Physis* (Basel, 1945). The opposition between "name" (*onoma*) and "work" or "reality" (*ergon*) has the same sense. Does the "name" of a thing express what it is "in reality"? Recall the discussion in the *Cratylus* of Plato about the names of the gods. The antithesis between "being" and "seeming" or between "truth" and "opinion," so central, as is well known, in the philosophical thought of Parmenides, belongs to the same series and possesses similar significance.

It must not be thought however that in the fifth century *logos* and *ergon* are always antithetical terms. Thucydides calls Pericles "Most eminent in speaking and in doing" (I, 139, 4), and Chirisophus approves of the behavior of Xenophon both because of what the latter says as well as because of what he does (*Anab.*, III, 1, 45).

enemy of persuasion: thanks to it the two girls who guide him on the road of truth get *Dikê* to consent to clear the way for him (frag. 1, 15–16). Empedocles, too, spoke of the "royal highway of persuasion" (frag. 133) and according to Plutarch (*Quaest. conv.* IX, 5) contrasted musical Persuasion with non-musical and silent Necessity; "the Graces hate unbearable *Anankê*," he used to say (frag. 116), ill-resigned perhaps to the barriers that Nature opposes to man's power. Democritus will prove no less a believer in the divine power of the word. "The word is often mightier for persuasion than gold," one of his passages (frag. 51) asserts. In another the opposition between *peithô* and *anankê* once more appears, the latter in the sense—political and not cosmic or "natural"—of "coercion": "He who employs encouragement and the persuasive word will be a more powerful prompter to virtue than he who uses the law and coercion" (frag. 181). The law (*nomos*) too can be violent and coercive, and thus it will be good only when it persuades: "only to those whom it persuades does it show its virtue" (frag. 248).

The persuasive power of the word is confined within the wall which *Bia* and *Anankê* erect around it. What things are by nature cannot change by the action of our *logos*. But what if what things "are" does not depend so much upon their nature, their *physis,* as upon what we agree that they "are," upon the *nomos* or law of our social existence? [76] It is true that in many aspects of reality convention will never have any power against nature, nor *nomos* against *physis:* say what we may, and agree upon what we may, gold will always be yellow. But does it not perhaps depend upon a tacit agreement or consent among men that gold is valuable? Undoubtedly there are many aspects of reality in which *nomos* defeats *physis*. This is the great, the dazzling discovery of the Sophists. This discovery of theirs is destined to fascinate them so much they will often misuse it unscrupulously. By means of persuasion the word of man can create new conventions; accordingly it can determine the essence of things. The persuasive word, as if it

[76]. Again I refer the reader to the excellent study by Heinimann, *Nomos und Physis.*

had the magic power of a charm or a spell, changes reality. It can no longer surprise us that Gorgias should give the name of *epôdê* to the persuasive word or that, with his master Corax, he should call rhetoric—his great invention—*peithous demiourgos*, "demiurge of persuasion" (Plato, *Gorg.*, 453a, 455a).

The Sophist doctrine of persuasion has its most original and careful exponent in Gorgias. In the Sicilian school of rhetoric, of Corax and Tisias, where Gorgias received his first formal instruction, one was taught to esteem probability more highly than truth, and by force of the word to make the little appear great and the great little (Plato, *Phaedrus*, 267a–b). Nothing so well illustrates the importance of persuasion in this school as an anecdote about these two Sicilian rhetors. Tisias says to Corax: "If you have taught me to persuade, then I persuade you not to charge me any fee for your instruction; and if you have not taught me, neither shall I pay you, for you taught me nothing." Corax twisted the argument in his favor, and the tribunal that was to judge them said as its only decision: "An evil crow [*korax:* crow] has laid a bad egg." [77] The "bad egg" would be Tisias, the pupil of Corax.

Educated in this school and endowed as well with a wonderful talent for oratory, Gorgias made persuasion the basis of his professional life and the hub of his own thought. Supreme means for success in persuasive action, the word "is a powerful sovereign, for with a very tiny and completely invisible body it performs the most divine works. It has in fact the power to take away fear, banish pain, inspire happiness and increase compassion" (*Enc. Hel.*, 8). Most accurately and significantly Gorgias compares the working of the word to the action of medicaments. In relation to the good order of the soul (*psychês taxis*), the word must have a *dynamis* or power wholly comparable to that possessed by well-compounded medicines (*pharmakôn taxis*) in relation to the nature of the body (EH, 14). This is so much the case that if *peithô*, the persuasion of the human word, must be contrasted to *bia*, the force or violence of men (EH, 6), as traditional wisdom

77. The anecdote probably comes from the Sicilian comedy. I have taken it from Nestle, p. 310.

teaches, it is no less true that she, *Peithô*, can also succeed in forcing the will of those who are the object of her influence. Soon we shall see how.

How does persuasion work? What happens in the mind of one whom the word has persuaded? With a phrase that may have come from Gorgias, Plato on one occasion calls rhetoric *psychagôgia,* the art of directing minds by means of speech. The orator must therefore be acquainted with the various "aspects" (*eidê*) which the minds of men display if he really is endeavoring to speak adequately to the character of each one of them (*Phaedrus,* 271c–d). Moreover, he will take very well into account the "occasion" (*kairos*) on which he is speaking (Gorgias, frag. 13 Diels); that is, the mood at that time of the person who is to be persuaded by his words. *Eidos* and *kairos* of the soul are, then, the two primary realities in the art of "psychagogy."

This with respect to the subject of persuasion, the hearer. As concerns the method, Gorgias implicitly resorts to three models: the "meteorologist," the "political orator," and the "philosopher." The "meteorologist"—with this word Gorgias is alluding, as is obvious, to the pre-Socratic "physiologists"—with his reasonings succeeds in driving everyday opinions about things from the mind and in replacing them with others in which what was previously incredible and invisible becomes obvious; the "political orator," for his part, delights and persuades public assemblies by the force of his argument, if the latter has been written according to the rules of art; the "philosopher," finally, shows in his discussions the swiftness and the subtlety of his thoughts and with them easily succeeds in changing in the mind of those who hear him their former trust (*pistis*) in some determined opinion (EH, 13).[78] Whoever seeks with his words "to engrave" persuasion in the mind of another must adhere to these three different models in his practice.

---

78. To what "philosophers" is Gorgias alluding? To the Eleatic, as G. Bux suspects ("Gorgias und Parmenides," *Hermes,* 76, 1941, 393–407), or to the cultivators of the Eristic school, as Diès and Nestle maintain (p. 326)?

It is not difficult to note that for Gorgias the convictions produced in their hearers by the meteorologist, the political orator, and the philosopher coincide in something fundamental: the three must be opinions (*doxai*) rather than objective truths, and in the three it is faith or trust (*pistis*) that causes them to be considered acceptable and true. In Greek, *peithô*, opinion, and *pistis*, belief, are words derived from the same root. This enables us to take one more step in the understanding of Gorgias' thought and to answer the second of the questions posed previously: what happens in the soul of the one persuaded?

The persuasive word, Gorgias thinks, acts upon the soul as do medicaments upon the body. "Just as some medicines eliminate one humor from the body, and other medicines another, and some free from disease while others take away life, so too do some words grieve, others cheer, others frighten, others inflame him who listens to them and others, finally, with effectively malign persuasion poison and bewitch the soul" (EH, 14). All of which is possible insofar as the word is technically able to instill some belief (*pistis*) in the mind of the hearer. "Rhetoric," trenchantly says Socrates to Gorgias in the Platonic dialogue of the same title, "must be the demiurge of persuasion; persuasion relating to a belief, not knowledge, about the just and the unjust" (*Gorg.*, 454e–455a). The rhetor, by his very nature, which demands manliness, daring, and a capacity for conjecture and divination (*Gorg.*, 463a; Isocrates, *c. soph.*, 17), and because of the education he has received, is a man more persuasive and more easily believed (*pithanôteros*) than the cultivators of the remaining techniques (*Gorg.*, 456c, 457a, 459a). Now then: why is man obliged to adhere to opinions and why must the latter be obtained by persuasion and maintained by belief?

The reply of Gorgias is radical, though insufficient. This happens, he finally tells us, because man is a limited and deficient being.

> If all men had memory of all past events and knowledge of the present and foreknowledge of the future, the word,

> even though it were similar, would not deceive as it now does. But we have no way to recall the past, to look deeply into the present and to divine the future. Therefore, regarding most problems, the majority offer the mind an instructive opinion [*doxan symboulon*]. But opinion is unsure and inconstant and hence casts those who have resort to it into unsure and inconstant misfortunes. (EH, 11)

Gorgias means that man cannot know reality with sufficient certainty; consequently he has to adhere, not to true knowledge, but to an opinion (*doxa*); it turns out, however, that opinion is insecure and leads one astray. In this case, what can man do if he wants to live with some security? Only this remains possible to him: to get one who knows more than he does to instill in him by persuasion an opinion "better" than his, in other words, for another and wiser man—the Sophist—to make him believe and trust in that which for his need is the most favorable thing. That belief in the opinion received will give his life the security and the foundation which it did not have before. The excellence of such an opinion will prevent him, moreover, from falling into misfortune (*atychia*). Thus it is that persuasion, paradoxically, comes to effect souls as violence (*bia*) and necessity (*ananké*) do (EH, 12). In short it might be said that the convention (*nomos*) created by the persuasive word has somehow become the nature (*physis*) of the man upon whom that word has come to act.

Persuasion is in a way "deceit" (*apaté*) (EH, 11), but advantageous and justifiable deceit (*dikaia apaté*) if it seeks the good of the man persuaded. Persuasion is also in some respect a "malady": Gorgias says that the contemplation of a beautiful work of sculpture "produces a sweet malady in the eyes," and that in the spectator "it awakens love and longing for things [*pragmata*] and persons [*sômatôn*]" (EH, 18). And does not listening to poetry—Gorgias is thinking above all of tragedy: another justifiable deceit (frag. 23)—perchance cause in the hearer "a thrill full of terror, a compassion which is shed as tears and a fierce anguish which takes pleasure in its own pain?" (EH, 9). The seduction of the soul by everything that is really capable of seduction disturbs, moves, impassions, and breeds a *pathos* which can almost be called a "malady," *nosos*. All this is equivalent to saying that the "justifiable deceit," the placing of human existence within a determined "convention" or *nomos*—even though such a "convention" be limited on occasion to two persons, the one who persuades and the one persuaded—has come to modify a *physis* artfully and technically. It is not false to the thought of Gorgias to say that according to him human *physis* could attain nobility and eminence only by the aid of a certain "malady," a certain "deceit," and a certain "sorcery." Now we well understand the ultimate scope of the metaphors that transform the persuasive word into "glad satiety," "charm," and "witchery."

But we have also heard that the persuasive word is a *pharmakon*, in the double sense, medicament and poison, of that Greek term: a "drug" by virtue of which the great law of Nature is fulfilled, as Gorgias understands it: the weaker should be dominated and led by the stronger (EH, 6). He who knows how to persuade is always the stronger and one who knows how to enslave others: "With this power—that which rhetoric bestows—you will make the physician your slave, and the trainer your slave; and the financier will soon realize that he has not financed for himself but for another, for you, who know how to speak and persuade the multitude," says Socrates to the Gorgias of the Platonic dialogue (*Gorg.*, 452e). The medicament of the persuasive word can be poison or remedy for other men, according to the intention with which it is used. Since that word modifies the *physis* of one who hears it, can it be therefore at the same time a medicine to cure the sick man? Is the Sophist doctrine of persuasion also the doctrine of a logotherapy in the most purely medical sense of this word?

The truth is that the Sophist movement had from its inception a close relationship to medicine, the prestige of which as a *technê*—if you will, as "technical knowledge"—was already great in Greece during the first half of the fifth century. It is moreover admissible to say, as does Zubiri, that "medicine was Sophism's great argument for the world." Protagoras resorts to medical experience in order to justify the relativistic themes of his work, "On the Truth." The taste of the same food, for example, may be one for the the man in good health and another for the sick man; what is sweet to the former is bitter to the latter. Each individual has his own sensations, and the quality of these is conditioned by the habitual state or "habit" (*hexis*) of health or illness. Hence, Protagoras concludes, it cannot be said that the sensation of the healthy man is "truer" than that of the sick man; to the latter "the bitter" is as real as "the sweet" to the former. The sensation is always "true." The physician therefore will not seek to convince the patient that his sensation is "false"; but with therapeutic remedies will try to convert the "habit" of the patient into another and better one, which will transform the feeling of sickness into a normal feeling no more "true" than the former.[79] This way of seeing things is to have a twofold result. As regards philosophy it will be maintained that thinking is, in a way, a type of feeling; whereupon "being" will come to mean "to be felt" (Zubiri). Philosophical thought thus very decidedly situates itself in the realm of sensation and opinion: the important thing will no longer be to have a "true" opinion but to have a "better" opinion. As for medicine, it will be thought that health and illness —the so-called modes of life—are "conventional" states or habits of human nature, not differing from one another because one corresponds more than the other to the "truth" and the "essence" of that nature, but because one of them, health, is "more advantageous," "more valuable" (*ameinôn, beltiôn*) than the other for the life of man.[80]

79. See Nestle, *Vom Mythos zum Logos,* pp. 269–70.
80. According to Th. Gomperz (*Die Apologie der Heilkunst,* 2d ed. Leipzig, 1910) the relations between Protagoras and medicine must not have ended there; the Sophist of Abdera was probably also the author of the work in the *Corpus Hippocraticum* which bears the title of *peri technês* or *de arte.* Gomperz's conjecture does not enjoy much credit today.

But more important to us now than this theoretical connection between the Sophists and medicine are the possible therapeutic consequences of the Sophistic doctrine of conjecture. There were in fact such connections. The comparison, from the pen of Gorgias, between persuasive speeches and medicaments was not a simple rhetorical gambit. A passage from Plato proves this beyond the shadow of doubt. Gorgias says to Socrates:

> If you knew everything, Socrates, you would see that it [rhetoric] embodies in itself and holds in sway all powers. I am going to give you a good proof of it. It has often occurred to me to accompany my brother [81] or other physicians to the house of some patient who was refusing a medicine or who would not allow himself to be treated by iron and fire; when the physician's admonitions were powerless I would persuade the patient with no other art than rhetoric. Let a rhetor and a physician go together to whatever city you will: if a discussion is begun in the assembly of the people or in any gathering to decide which of the two will be elected as physician, I declare that the physician will disappear and the orator will be preferred, if it so please him. (*Gorg.*, 456b)

Let us abstain for a moment from the well-aimed reply of Socrates and consider another testimony even more valuable, relating to the Sophist Antiphon.[82] "During the time in which he was devoting himself to poetry," says the Pseudo-Plutarch (*Vit. X orat.*, I, 18), "he founded an art to cure griefs, analo-

---

81. Gorgias was a brother of the physician Herodicus of Leontini (*Gorg.*, 448b).
82. In the final decades of the fifth century there were in Athens probably three Antiphons, whom later tradition frequently mixed up and confused: a Sophist, a political orator of the oligarchy, and an author of tragedies. Philosophers have discussed the personality and the work of each one of them at length. See: J. Stenzel, "Antiphon," *RE* Suppl. Bd. 4, cols. 33–43; Nestle, pp. 395–400; L. Gernet, *Antiphon* (Paris, "Les Belles Lettres," 1954). There are those who admit the existence of only one Antiphon (Joel, for example), as opposed to those who assert that there were two (Nestle), and even three (Heinimann).

gous to that one which among physicians serves as a basis for the treatment of diseases; in Corinth, near the agora, he arranged a place with a sign, in which he announced himself as able to treat the grief-stricken [*tous lypoumenous*] by means of discourses; and informing himself of the causes [of the affliction] he unburdened and consoled [*paremytheito*] the patients. But judging that this occupation [*technê*] was beneath him he addressed himself to rhetoric." [83] Philostratus tells us that the performance of certain "soothing" or "consoling recitations" [*nêpentheis akroaseis*] won the Sophist the sobriquet of "Nestor" (Diels, A 6). We know, finally, that Antiphon was an interpreter of portents and dreams (*teratoskopos kai oneirokritês*), according to the statements of Suidas, Hermogenes, Diogenes Laertius, and Lucian, who are in agreement on this (Diels, A 1, 2, 5, and 7).[84]

So, therefore, that initial "persuasive" or "cheering speech" of which Nestor and Patroclus made use in the Homeric world has become a technique with Gorgias and Antiphon. By verbal persuasion patients confidently accept medical treatment (Gorgias), and certain grief-stricken persons, now precisely classified as sick (*kamnontas,* the text of the Pseudo-Plutarch says), receive relief and consolation (Antiphon). How and to what point was this possible? And above all how did those two Sophists interpret their unquestionably psychotherapeutic attitude?

We already know what would be fundamental in the possible reply of Gorgias. The Sicilian Sophist places in contrast to his *Eulogy of Helen* the anomalous affections caused by the gods and the "human maladies" (*anthrôpinon nosêma*). These, he says, are a misfortune free of guilt (*atychia*), not in-

83. The verb *paramytheomai,* which so expressively alludes to the narrative word or *mythos,* at the same time means "to alleviate" and "to console." It has seemed to me that its sense in this case would remain more clear by combining the two definitions.

84. In addition to the sources cited here, I refer the reader to W. Kranz and W. Leibbrand, "Der erste Arzt für seelische Leiden," *Allg. Ztschr. für Psych.,* 1943–44, and to the book of W. Leibbrand, *Der göttliche Stab des Aeskulap,* 3d ed. (Salzburg, 1939).

volving moral responsibility on the part of the one who suffers them (EH, 19). How can the professional rhetor be a better physician against them than the practitioner of medicine? Gorgias might answer thus: because verbal persuasion, the medicament of the persuasive word, not only dominates the will but can also modify the entire *physis*, body and soul, of the man upon whom it acts. Persuasion therefore will make the healthy man believe that the rhetor is a more able therapist than the physician, and will be able to effect the cure of the sick man by modifying his upset *physis*. All the more if to the medicament of his word the rhetor knows how to add medicines that act upon the body.

It is worthwhile to explain the objection of Socrates. Here is the outline of his argument: a) the rhetor is more persuasive than the physician before the multitude, that is, before those who do not know; before those who know, he could not be; b) the rhetor, in the first place, does not know medicine; in persuading the multitude, he is an ignorant man speaking before ignorant men; c) rhetoric then does not need to know the reality of things; the persuasion which it has invented is sufficient for it to appear to ignorant men wiser than the wise; d) this conclusion then is necessary: either the rhetor who is trying to cure must know medicine as an art, that is, by knowing how to do things according to what the medicaments and the reality of the patient "are," or rhetoric is nothing but a crude and conventional empiricism, with no other feature than the mere pleasure or the pure advantage of the one who practices it, like any other of the several activities that "seek the pleasurable without caring for the best" (*Gorg.*, 459a–465a). "Cuisine," Socrates will later say,

> seemed to me to be a routine and not an art, unlike medicine, and I gave this reason: that medicine when it treats a patient, has begun by studying nature and knows why it works as it does, and can give a reason for all this; while cuisine, whose endeavor seeks merely pleasure, goes toward its goal without art, without having studied the

nature of pleasure or its cause, at random in everything so to speak, lacking calculation, preserving only through routine practice the memory of what is ordinarily done and thus trying to achieve pleasure. (501a)

Near the end of his life, in the *Philebus,* Plato will again set forth his old idea. The subject is to know what the "power of the dialogue" consists of. The question is important if one thinks that "dialectic" has its basis and its source in the "dialogue" or *dialegein.* Persuasion or dialectic; this is the problem. What to think about it? Young Protarchus has heard Gorgias say time and again that "the art of persuading far surpasses the others, for it subjects all to its rule voluntarily and not by force." Socrates, more prudent and profound, will solemnly declare it to be beyond doubt that "knowledge of being, of true reality, always identical by nature" is the true reason for that eminent *dynamis* of the dialogue (*Phil.,* 58a–b). Against the shifting power of the opinions that persuasion instills, Plato raises up the supreme and unshakeable power of the truth which the intelligence knows.

In summary: the therapeutic rhetoric of Gorgias would consider only the "opinion" of the patient; the technical cures of the expert in medicine adhere, on the other hand—or at least attempt to adhere—to the "truth" of what health, disease, and the nature of the patient "are." Above the persuasive *logos* should be the noetic and scientific *logos.* Gorgias himself, the real Gorgias, will find himself obliged to think thus when in his *Apology of Palamedes* he endeavors to persuade his hearers "not with words of compassion but with the greatest evidence of the just and with demonstration of the truth" (AP, 33). But what if the technical knowledge of the physician is added to the persuasion of the rhetorician? In other words, what if the mythical or persuasive *logos,* the *logos pithanos,* were as indispensable in the life of man as the dialectic *logos?* In this case would not Socrates and Plato have to modulate their judgments? The next chapter will give us the brilliant reply of both.

Let us now take up the thought of Antiphon; let us investigate with some care how the author of the work, "The Truth" (*Alêtheia*), was able to understand and explain his psychotherapeutic treatments in Corinth. Antiphon consoled and relieved, by means of the word, patients whose dominant symptom was sorrow, grief (*lypê*). What could he think of this practice of his? It is not too daring to suppose that the point of departure of his doctrine must have been the antithesis between *nomos* (the law: the conventional, the established and prescribed, the "legal") and *physis* (nature, the original and radical, the genuine and spontaneous, the truly "natural" and "real" part of human life) [85], an antithesis already foreshadowed in Greek literature prior to the publication of the above work by Antiphon and very vigorously and systematically developed in the latter. Translating the thought of Gorgias into the language of so famous a contrast [86] he would say the following: by means of the persuasion of the rhetorician the patient, painfully and helplessly situated within his own *nomos*, and unable to escape from it alone, succeeds in placing himself in another *nomos* more favorable than the previous one and more conformable to his own *physis*. An intuitive knowledge of the "aspect," "type," or *eidos* of the soul of the patient and of his temporary condition or *kairos* might enable the rhetorician to act according to art in his persuasive task. To this knowledge of the *eidos* and the *kairos* of the soul of the patient—I am following the text of Pseudo-Plutarch—Antiphon adds a new requirement: the knowledge of the cause (*aitia*) of the affliction. With this he will draw closer to the intellectual demand of Socrates, Plato, and Aristotle, according to which a human activity cannot be called "art" (*technê*) un-

---

85. Bear all those meanings in mind in order to understand with some accuracy what those two terms were for a Greek of the fifth century. As for the concept of *physis*, see, besides *Nomos und Physis*, by Heinimann, the works of H. Diller, "Der griechische Naturbegriff," *Neue Jahrbücher für Antike und deutsche Bildung 2* (1939), 241–57, and of K. Deichgräber, "Die Stellung des griechischen Arztes zur Natur," *Die Antike 15* (1939), 116–38.

86. Gorgias, as we have seen, lives and acts within it.

less it is based upon knowledge of the "why" of that which is done. The Sophist Antiphon, however, will say something more.

Directly influenced by Eleatic philosophy, Antiphon is less a relativist than are Protagoras and Gorgias: very express indeed is the opposition that he establishes between thought (*gnômê*) and sensation (*aisthêsis*), and between truth (*alêtheia*) and opinion (*doxa*). But the decisive factor in him may well be, as I have said, his bold appeal to the *nomos-physis* antithesis. The *nomos* is the product of human convention (*homologêsis*); its precepts are arbitrary, artificial, as if superadded (*epitheta*); hence it is opposed to the free development of the *physis* of man. Now all this is ultimately harmful. *Physis* has deep within it a final and inexorable "necessity" (*anankê physeôs*), which is of such a nature that obeying it, following the impulses of Nature herself, causes man to feel joyously free. "Enjoy nature, laugh, leap, and do not consider anything to be shameful!" says a character of Aristophanes (*Clouds,* 1078) after having invoked the *anankê physeôs* and surely influenced by the same mentality that the thought of Antiphon expresses. It is true that man with his whims and conventions can transgress the commands of that "necessity of nature"; the human being is in a way independent of his *physis*, but he who transgresses them will have to bear the consequences, for the *anankê* of *physis* is inexorable. The expedient—to do the expedient thing (*to xympheron*) should be the supreme rule of life—consists then in being faithful to *physis* and in freeing the latter from the disturbing coercions of *nomos*. The devaluation of the *nomos*, from the time when Pindar termed its right application *nomos pharmakôn* or "law of medicaments" (*Nem.*, III, 55) and saw Zeus behind the "law" or *nomos* of the city (*Pyth.*, II, 86), is extremely evident. Something serious has happened in Greek life to produce that impressive change.

But in the thought of Antiphon is there not perhaps an internal contradiction and a dangerous threat of hedonism and libertinism? Necessity (*anankê physeôs*) sets man free and binds and enslaves for him what is free convention (*nomos*) in his life. How is this possible? And will not surrender to the free spontaneity of Nature, rebellion against the *nomos*, lead as in Aristophanes' comedy to the most individualistic and shameless licentiousness? Antiphon appears to have suspected this objection, which Democritus, even without having expressly formulated it, will perhaps try to overcome by distinguishing a true *anankê* and a merely apparent one in the web of men's behavior, and by asserting the human need to add reasonable "conventions" to spontaneous "impulses."

Let us now leave Democritus' solution and take up our problem: the psychotherapeutic curing of sorrows and afflictions of morbid character. Man can act against the necessity of his *physis*, and this brings him pain; but he can also act in accordance with that necessity and this affords him pleasure. This latter is what is expedient (*to xympheron*). But are there not perchance in life two types of expediencies: those which correspond to *physis* and those which are ruled by *nomos*? Antiphon thinks so: "The expedient, insofar as laws prescribe it, is a bond of nature; it is free, on the other hand, if it depends on her. Therefore, according to right opinion, it is not true that things distressing [*ta algynonta*] aid nature more than do things pleasing [*ta euphrainonta*]; consequently, neither must it be true that things painful [*ta lypounta*] are more expedient than things pleasurable [*ta hêdonta*]. The truly expedient must not do harm, but be advantageous" (Diels, B 44, 4).

An important paragraph. In it Antiphon throws overboard the old teaching of Aeschylus: that *pathei mathos* which assumed the need to suffer in order to know and therefore to give excellence to the *physis*. He establishes moreover two classes of expediencies: the true, pertaining to the *physis*, and the apparent and false which the *nomos* prompts or imposes; the former are always helpful and the latter are ultimately harmful. He contrasts, finally, two pairs of affections: distressing-pleasing and painful-pleasurable. What meaning does this stylistic show have? Diels [87] thought that the first pair of concepts might have a corporeal sense and the second a psychical

---

87. *Intern. Monatschrift*, 11 (1916), 93.

sense. This Heinimann denies because the counterposition possesses the formal structure of the rhetorical games that Prodicus had taught men to use; but he finds himself obliged to concede that under the verbal cleverness there is here something else, for *algynonta* ("the distressing") has reference, in contrast with *lypounta* ("the painful"), to pain immediately felt and to which the *physis* reacts; that is, to the pain which we are still accustomed to call "physical." It might be said that "the distressing" is the reaction of the *physis* to what is directly disadvantageous for it, and that "the painful" is the state produced by that which, seeming to be advantageous—being *xympheron* according to the *nomos*—is ultimately harmful instead. Perhaps the distinction of Antiphon may not be very far removed from that which Plutarch will establish between "pains caused by nature" (*lypoun physei*) and "pains according to opinion" (*lypoun doxê*) (*peri euthym.*, c. 17).

Be this as it may, the important thing is to know how the painful can be eliminated from life. Antiphon believes that for this purpose there is a technique (*technê alypias*); moreover, he practices that *technê* by informing himself of the causes of the affliction and speaking to the patient accordingly. Verbal persuasion, acting according to the causes, succeeds in eliminating pain from the mind: the thought and the word of the curative rhetorician, his *logos*, set in order and rationalize the psychic and physical life of the sufferer. "In all men," another passage from Antiphon says, "the intelligence [*gnômê*] rules the body both in respect to health and illness as in all the rest" (frag. 2 Diels). For the coward "illness is a holiday, for thus he does not go to work" (frag. 57); but for him who rules his life reasonably, illness is an occasion to master the body and put it in order by doing the expedient; ultimately rationalizing it and naturalizing it at one and the same time, on the one hand by subjecting it to the dictates of intelligence and on the other by bringing it back to what is by nature best for it. A judgment of Stenzel regarding Antiphon's doctrine of the reality of human life can also be applied to the problem of healing: "There is not in this attitude a naturalization of the logos or a rationalization of nature, but the undivided unity of a reality that is for that very reason psycho-physical."[88] Upon that "undivided unity" the word of the rhetorician must work by pointing out to the sufferer the way to the rationalization and the naturalization of his life and by moving him through persuasion to follow it.

But would this be possible if the rhetorician did not give to the *physis* of the patient a new *nomos*, a new vital "convention" believingly accepted by him and more advantageous to his life, more "natural," than that in which he was living in pain and sickness? In other words: is it possible for the *physis* of man to live without conventions, without *nomoi*? Is not man indeed a being physically and essentially nomic or conventional? Is not the liberation from the *nomoi* which Antiphon proposes as a means to the health and well-being of the human race, life "according to nature," *kata physin*, actually a new *nomos* different from that which traditionally had ruled in the Greek city and been extolled by Pindar and Solon? The obstinate hostility of the Sophist against "convention" prevents him from seeing this. Democritus, on the other hand, will succeed in seeing it and saying it.[89]

Democritus too appeals to the efficacy of the *logos*—in this case, the scientific *logos*, of reasoning—for the treatment of affliction: "It expels by means of reasoning [*logismôi*] the rebellious grief from a benumbed mind," says one of his maxims (frag. 290 Diels). Wisdom frees the mind of passions, as medi-

[88]. J. Stenzel, col. 36.
[89]. The work of Antiphon—"incunabulum of Attic philosophy," it has been called—clearly shows what today everyone admits: that the relations between Sophism and philosophy in the strict sense are considerably more complex and finely shaded than the picture painted by Plato would lead one to think. With respect to the themes treated here, and in addition to the works of Nestle, Jaeger, Th. Gomperz, Stenzel, and Heinimann already indicated, the following bibliography may be consulted: A. Diès, "Notes sul l'HELENES ENKHOMION de Gorgias," *Revue de philol.* 37 (1913), 192–206; H. Gomperz, *Sophistik und Rhetorik* (Leipzig, 1912); W. Süss, *Ethos. Studien zur älteren griechischen Rhetorik* (Leipzig, 1910); W. Luther, *Wahrheit und Lüge im ältesten Griechentum* (Leipzig, 1935); M. Untersteiner, *I Sofisti* (Turin, 1940) and *Sofisti, Testimonianze e frammenti* (Florence, 1949).

cine cures the diseases of the body (frag. 31). Democritus moreover knows that there are three types of illnesses: maladies "of the house" (*oikou*), "of the way of living" (*biou*), and "of the body" (*skêneos*) (frag. 288). A brilliant concept, this one of *nosos biou* or "malady of the way of living"; those in Corinth who used to come to the consulting office of Antiphon must have been suffering from it, and many of those who today consult psychotherapists suffer from it. But for what purpose do they consult them? So that the physician by means of his diagnostic technique and his word may rid the *physis* of the patient of his attachment to every kind of *nomoi* and may teach him to rule freely over the latter? To act, in short, in accordance with the doctrines of Antiphon?

Democritus is more profound. In man as in all living beings the drives of nature are active; but a drive—the sexual, for example—is not truly human unless it has been shaped by *nomoi* or conventions, such as those of thinking that procreation is advantageous (frag. 278) or, on the contrary, that it is better to have few children (frag. 276). In a very general and clear way fragment 33 asserts this: "Nature and education are analogous things; education transforms men, but by that transformation it creates nature [*physiopoiei*]." Hence it is that the wise man should be able to distinguish among the different "needs" (*anankai*) of nature. There are some indeed very deep and inexorable, such as that of living, and in the case of these it is foolish not to obey (frag. 289); but there are also some that are superficial and apparent, and among them it is necessary to distinguish which are advantageous and which are harmful (frags. 223, 234, 235), in order to seat them more and more deeply in nature by means of the educative and "physiopoietic" efficacy of reasonable *nomoi* in the case of the advantageous needs and to eliminate them energetically and aggressively in the case of the harmful ones. "To strive against one's [own] spirit is a difficult thing; but it is characteristic of prudent men to win the victory," says Democritus (frag. 236).

It appears certain that Democritus practiced medicine. A note from Aulus Gellius—spurious according to Diels, acceptable according to Delatte [90]—presents him as the author of a book on the cure of disease by music, but it is not possible to determine whether the sage of Abdera put into practice his precept to banish afflictions from the mind through reasoning. In any case it is certain that in his writings there were ideas capable of explaining verbal psychotherapy, with its real possibilities and its indubitable limits, far better than do the Sophist doctrines of Gorgias and Antiphon. But much more broadly, subtly, and profoundly than the pre-Socratic and Sophist philosophers one who towers over all of them is to speak to us of the therapy of the word: the divine Plato.

90. *Les conceptions de l'enthousiasme*, pp. 74–78. Democritus is more a philosopher and more traditional than Antiphon. His attitude toward *enthousiasmos* and *mania*—at once traditional and "scientific," since it is based on his atomism—shows this very clearly. It appears very probable that Democritus, as Delatte supposes, must also have given an atomistic interpretation to the medicinal action of music. For the therapeutic use of the latter in classical Antiquity, see the work of L. Edelstein, *Greek Medicine in its Relation to Religion and Magic*, previously mentioned. The relation between rhetoric and music has been recently studied by W. Gurlitt ("Musik und Rhetorik," *Helicon*, 5, 1944, 67 ff.) and A. Schmitz (*Die Bildlichkeit der wortgebundenen Musik Johann Sebatian Bachs*, Mainz, 1950).

Chapter 3

The Platonic Rationalization of the Charm

In Vienna in the year 1925 a book of unquestionable importance in the history of contemporary medicine was published.[1] At the beginning of its text a passage from the *Charmides* of Plato (156d–157a) was printed, that in which Socrates says that he has learned from a Thracian, a disciple of Zamolxis, that the maladies of the body cannot be cured without treating before and above all the soul. "But the soul," the passage there quoted ends by saying, "is cured by certain charms." The discernment of the one who was wise enough to choose that passage was undoubtedly great: the pages that follow will prove this conclusively. But his insufficiency was as great as his discernment, for the truly inspired and decisive element in the thought of Plato on the subject appears elsewhere in the same dialogue—an insufficiency, it should be added, never remedied by the many physicians who have since then copied those prophetic words of the Athenian philosopher.

Nor have philosophers studied in a fully satisfactory manner the Platonic idea of the charm or conjuration (*epôdê*): not the acute Welcker, nor the conscientious Pfister, nor Heim in his collection of texts,[2] nor authors such as Boyancé and Dodds who have written subsequently in a more or less direct and detailed way about the attitude of Plato toward the *epôdê*.

It appears therefore that a study of this problem from a twofold point of view, historico-cultural and medical, can still throw some light on Plato's knowledge of anthropology and

1. *Psychogenese und Psychotherapie körperlicher Symptome*, ed. by O. Schwarz (Vienna, 1925).
2. Heim, "Incantamenta magica Graeca et Latina," *Jahrb f. Philol.*, Suppl. *19*. The works of Welcker and Pfister have been reviewed on previous pages.

his personal ideas about the curative action of the physician.

I. The word *epôdê* and those related to it—the verbs *epadô, katepadô,* and *exepadô,* the adjective and the noun *epôdos*—are used in the writings of Plato, if my count is not in error, no less than 52 times [3]: 20 in the *Charmides,* 2 in the *Gorgias,* 1 in the *Meno,* 2 in the *Euthydemus,* 1 in the *Banquet,* 5 in the *Phaedo,* 4 in the *Republic,* 1 in the *Phaedrus,* 2 in the *Theaetetus,* and 14 in the *Laws.* This enumeration shows quite clearly that the idea of the *epôdê* was present in the mind of Plato throughout his whole life as a writer, from the dialogues of his youth to those of his extreme old age. But it is still curious that the greatest frequency of use corresponds to one of his first works, the *Charmides,* and to the one thought to be his last, the *Laws.* We shall presently see the relation that exists between these initial and final conceptions of the charm.

But the need to consider chronologically the Platonic view of the *epôdê* must be harmonized at once with another need, no less important, dependent upon the varying sense in which Plato uses the word. There are occasions on which the philosopher, in a traditional and direct way, limits himself to denoting by it the charms or magical conjurations which the Greek people had been practicing since prehistoric times. The word is in such cases much more denominative or descriptive than interpretative, even when its concrete meaning is not totally free from a value judgment, positive at times and negative at others. On the other hand there are passages in which the interpretative intention is evident. The term is not used then in its direct and traditional sense but with a new metaphorical or analogical meaning. In consequence it will be necessary to study separately these ways of using the word *epôdê* and to analyze subsequently what it means in the two dialogues in which the constructive effort of Plato is most conclusive, the *Charmides* and the *Laws.*

From the *epôdê* with which the sons of Autolycus heal Ulysses' wound on, mention of this therapeutic rite is frequent

[3]. The compilation offered in Ast's Lexicon is incomplete.

in Greek literature; recall what was said in the previous chapter. It concerns, as we know, a verbal formula of magical character, of variable content according to the case, recited or sung in the presence of the patient to bring about his cure. *Epôdê*, consequently, means conjuration, charm, incantation, or spell: "conjuration" when a commanding or coercive intention is predominant in the rite, "charm" when the preponderant intention is beseeching or imploring.

Plato alludes at times with very strict sobriety to these traditional *epôdai*; for example, when he speaks of how midwives are able to excite or relieve the pains of childbirth by the recitation of charms (*Theaet.*, 149c), or when he lists the various therapeutic measures of the Greek physician: medicaments, cauteries, incisions, and charms, *epôdai* (*Rep.*, IV, 426b). To a mere listing of magical practice is added in other instances the expression of an explicit attitude of moral and intellectual reproach. This occurs in Book II of the *Republic*: in his skillful plea on behalf of unjust living Adeimantus mentions "the charlatans and fortune-tellers who go about knocking at the doors of the rich and convince them that they have received from the gods the power to efface by means of conjurations performed amid merriment and feasts any sin that they or their ancestors may have committed" (*Rep.*, II, 364b).[4] The attack upon the magical *epôdai* is still more harsh in the final books of the *Laws*. Those who deceive and have contempt for men "by claiming that they can evoke the souls of the dead and by promising to seduce even the gods, bewitching them with sacrifices, prayers, and conjurations, *kai epôdais*" (*Laws*, X, 909b) are sentenced to solitary confinement for life in the central prison, and the fortune-tellers (*mantis*) and interpreters of portents (*teratoskopos*) who are reputed to cause harm by infernal invocations, conjurations (*epôdais*), and other sorcery are condemned to death (*Laws*, XI, 933d).

---

4. The ability of mania to efface guilts and ills of hereditary character is also mentioned, but with a tone of reproach, in *Phaedrus*, 244e. The passages from the *Republic* will be taken from the translation by J. M. Pabón and M. Fernández Galiano (*Platón. La República*, Madrid, 1949).

With equal explicitness and unanimity other passages in Plato refer to the magical *epôdê;* but there in one way or another the metaphorical or analogical intention that we shall study in the next section is hinted at. This occurs in the allusion to the charm made in the *Laws,* X, 906b: the "flattering words and enchanting prayers" which are alluded to here are both charms in the strict sense as well as natural means of seduction. And, in the *Symposium,* no less evident is the endeavor to remove the *epôdê* from the turbid and reprehensible realm of superstition and imposture when Socrates includes it among the several forms of the demonic (*to daimonion*): divination, sacrifices, initiations, charms, fortune-telling, and magic (*Symposium,* 201e–203a). As a demonic process the *epôdê* is one of the means for the mutual communication between gods and men. In this case can it be declared absolutely wicked?

A page from the *Euthydemus* boldly leads us into the field of the metaphorical or analogical utilization of the term. Socrates proposes in effect a precise, dichotomous classification of the art of charms: in its strictest sense that art consists of charming snakes, tarantulas, scorpions, other animals, and diseases; in another sense it is that of the makers of speeches (*logopoioi*) and is addressed to judges, to members of the Assembly, and to the multitudes in order to charm and calm them (*Euthyd.,* 290a). The word of the skilled orator is then a cause of enchantment or sorcery (*kêlêsis*), and therefore its art can be said to be divine, inspired by the gods (289e).[5] Hence the term *epôdê* can be legitimately applied to human activities very different from the magical treatment of wounds and diseases. This, as we know, is what not a few writers of the fifth century had already done.

The use that Plato makes of this literary discovery is not small. On the most varied occasions and for the most widely

5. In the text taken as a whole there is, as L. Méridier observes in his edition (*Les Belles Lettres,* Paris, 1949), a small contradiction. After stating that the art of speeches is a part of the art of charms, the statement that "it is hardly inferior to it" (289e) is made as though it were distinct. The sense is: the art of speeches and that of charms are parts of the same whole, and one of those parts is hardly inferior to the other.

differing reasons the characters of his dialogues apply the term *epôdê* to the psychologically effective word, to virtually or actually persuasive verbal expression. In the *Gorgias* during an impassioned defense of the law of the strongest Callicles calls "charmers" those who with softly seductive speeches persuade children that the just and the beautiful consist in having no more than others (484a).[6] Meno, for his part, maintains that Socrates fills him with perplexity by the "extreme charm" of his dialectic (*Men.*, 80a): dialectic is thus called *epôdê*. Socrates himself in the *Phaedrus* after having alluded ironically to the rhetoric art of various Sophists extolls the verbal power of the "colossus of Calcedon"—the Sophist Thrasymachus—able to infuriate a multitude and then, once the furious were subjected to his charms, to calm them (267d). No less clear is the non-magical sense of the *epôdê* in the *Theaetetus* when Socrates, after having expressly recalled the *epôdai* of midwives, designates his personal art of persuading with the word "maieutic," the art of midwifery, and tells his disciple that with it he enchants and bewitches him (157c). And this is how one may correctly understand the proposal to convert into an *epôdê* the charge that in the *Republic* attempts to prove the harmful effect of poetry: "so long as poetry has not justified itself we must, as it bewitches us, listen to it with the reasoning that we have made into a kind of charm to free ourselves from succumbing to a love more fitting to children and common men" (*Rep.*, X, 608a).

The meaning that *epôdê* has in the *Phaedo* deserves a paragraph to itself. The fear of death is at heart a childish fear, asserts Cebes after the argument of Socrates. Therefore, concludes Socrates, we must daily charm or enchant ourselves until our charm has extinguished that fear in us (77e). It is necessary then to seek at all costs an effective enchanter or

---

6. Such a task of persuasion would be useless in the case of the truly strong man: that man will rebel against false education, "casting down our writings, our sorceries, our charms, all our laws contrary to nature" (*Gorg.*, 484a).

charmer (*agathon epôdon*) against such terrors,[7] or, what may perhaps be more dependable among intelligent men, for each to become his own enchanter (78a). However, whether the first or the second be the case, what shall the text of the charm be? Through the mouth of the dying Socrates Plato, in the final pages of the dialogue, gives his answer: it is a myth, the long and complex myth of the destiny of souls, a myth in which men who are customarily called "prudent" or "of good sense" (*noun echontes*) perhaps will not believe, but men capable of daring will. "Beautiful is this venture indeed and in this type of belief there is as it were an enchanting of oneself," is Socrates' final judgment (144d). The myth, a beautiful and persuasive tale, acts as an *epôdê* against the noxious childishness of the fear of death.

The *epôdê*, which began as a conjuration or magical charm, has become reasoning or a tale against error or against harmful emotions. What is the nature of that semantic shift? Is it a simple metaphor, as Boyancé[8] and Dodds[9] assert, or something more important and profound?

To answer this question adequately let us begin by affirming the existence of a continuous transition between metaphor and intrinsic analogy. A genuine metaphor is always something more than an arbitrary verbal likening of two realities completely different from one another; thus when Jorge Manrique metaphorically calls human lives "rivers that flow down into the sea that is death," his expression supposes that between the reality of human life and the reality of a flowing river, as men see them, there is a real and not purely arbitrary relation. I would say, reducing the question to a simple formula, that the metaphor is an analogy in which the role of the speaker is

---

7. Socrates of course could excellently fill the bill; but Cebes and Simias are obliged to think of another because the philosopher is going to leave them.
8. *Le culte des Muses*, p. 36: "l'usage même métaphorique du mot *epôdê*."
9. P. 226. Dodds (*The Greeks and the Irrational*) speaks literally of a "metaphorical sense."

predominant and the analogy a metaphor in which the role of the subject itself is predominant; any example can serve to convince us of this, hence also of the use that Plato makes of the word *epôdê*.[10] An analysis of the *Charmides* and the *Laws* will present us with evidence for this.

II. Upon his return from the battle of Potidaea Socrates meets young Charmides in the gymnasium of Taureas and agrees to a request to cure him of the headache from which he is suffering. Socrates in fact knows an effective remedy against headaches: a certain plant, to which it is necessary to add an *epôdê*, a charm. To explain to the lad the power or virtue of this charm, he recalls to him that good physicians always treat the maladies of organs by ministering as well, with a suitable regimen, to the whole of the body, *diaita epi pan to sôma*.[11] Accordingly the application of the charm obeys this same principle, although carrying it to its ultimate consequences.

> I learned it [says Socrates] in the army from a Thracian physician, one of those pupils of Zamolxis who, they say, make men immortal. This Thracian told me that the Greek physicians are right in so saying; but Zamolxis, our king, who is a god—he added—teaches that just as it is not right to treat the eyes without treating the head, or the head without treating the body, so neither can the body be treated without treating the soul, and this is the reason why physicians among the Greeks are powerless against the majority of diseases, for they ignore the whole—with the malaise of which it is impossible for a single part to be—toward which their care should be directed. For

10. For the problem of the analogy and the metaphor, see Ortega y Gasset, *Obras completas* (Madrid, 1946–47), *1*, 448–51; *2*, 379–92; *3*, 372–75; and *4*, 256–61; B. Snell, "Gleichnis, Vergleich, Metaphor, Analogie," *Die Entdeckung des Geistes;* and my study "Poesía, ciencia y realidad," *Palabras menores* (Barcelona, 1952).

11. In *Laws*, X, 902d, Plato will emphasize correspondingly the importance of caring for the part: "Will a physician charged with treating the whole [*holon*] and who is willing and able to care for the greater aggregates, but neglects the parts and the details, ever see the whole [*to pan*] in good condition?"

everything, he said, the good as well as the bad, for the body and for the entire man, springs from the soul and flows from it as do the eyes from the body; because of which it is the soul whom, before all and above all (*kai prôton kai malista*), it is necessary to treat if one seeks the well-being of the head and the whole body. But the soul, my dear friend, he said, is treated with certain charms [*epôdais tisin*]. (*Charm.*, 156d-157a).

What do these charms able to cure the soul consist of? Through the mouth of the Thracian and of Socrates Plato gives a brief and clear reply: such charms are "beautiful discourses," *tous logous einai tous kalous.* "Through them temperance, *sôphrosynê*, is born in souls and once it has been engendered and is present, it is then easy to afford health to the head and to the rest of the body" (157a).[12]

The first statement in the reply merely repeats once more what we have been told in the preceding section: that beautiful speeches, speeches well embellished and able to persuade, are *epôdai*, charms of the soul. The second statement on the other hand adds an important new factor inasmuch as it reveals to us the thought of Plato about the psychological action of these metaphorical or analogical *epôdai* which are pertinent or beautiful speeches; that action consists in producing *sôphrosynê*.[13] This poses for Socrates the problem of knowing and stating precisely what is the virtue itself to which the Greeks gave so fair a name.

But before acquainting ourselves with the result of this

12. It is not possible to express in a single Spanish word the ensemble of intellectual, ethical, and aesthetic elements that the Greek concept of *sôphrosynê* embraces. To say "temperance," with the traditional enumeration of the cardinal virtues, is not sufficient, nor is it enough to say "serenity." The other modern languages meet with the same impossibility. Hence I have decided to use the Greek term without translation.

13. Pindar had already said (*Nem.*, IV, 1-6) that *euphrosyna* is the best physician for lasting woes: "songs, the wise daughters of the Muses, know how to enchant [*thelxan*] them with the soft caress of their hand, and hot water does not give our limbs as much lightness as do praises sung to the notes of the lyre." The comparison between the action of the word and the effect of the massage and the thermal bath is obvious.

investigation it will be well to take up in order the several suggestions of the Thracian follower of Zamolxis with respect to the right use of the charm against headaches. There appear to be three principal ones: 1. The charm and the vegetable medicament must be used together: for the plant to be a remedy (*pharmakon*) the charm must be added to it (155e); a very widespread error now among men, it is said subsequently, is to try to be separately physicians of the soul and the body (157b). 2. The performance of the charm must be prior to the administration of the medicine: "without the charm, the plant is of no avail" (155e); "let no one persuade you to treat his head if first he has not presented his soul for you to cure it with the charm" (157b). 3. The charm therefore cannot work if the patient has not "presented" or "offered" his soul (*paraschein*) to the one who is to treat it therewith: "And if you are willing, in accord with the provisions of the foreigner, first to present your soul to be enchanted by the charms of the Thracian I shall give you the medicine for your head; if not, dear Charmides, I do not know what I can do for you" (157c).[14]

The therapeutic *epôdê*, in summary, is a *logos kalos*, a "beautiful speech"; it takes effect by producing *sôphrosynê* in the soul; consequently the possession of *sôphrosynê* is a prior condition for the curative working of the *epôdê*. What then is *sôphrosynê*? Does Charmides already possess it in his soul, or is it rather necessary to provide him with it by means of the charm? "If *sôphrosynê* is already in you in sufficient measure you need neither the charms of Zamolxis nor those of Abaris the Hyperborean, and I can give you at once the medicament for your head; but if you think that you lack some of it, you must submit yourself to the charm before the administration of the medicament" (158b-c). And if *sôphrosynê* already exists in the soul of Charmides will the young man be able to express clearly and precisely what it is?

14. It is possible to add a fourth admonition, stated in the *Republic:* if the patient will not give up an unwholesome way of life because of waywardness neither the medicaments nor the *epôdai* will be of any use (*Rep.*, IV, 425e–426a).

The body of the dialogue is a reply to these three questions. In his colloquy with Charmides and Critias Socrates tries to find out what *sôphrosynê* is, whether it is present in the soul of Charmides before the charm is resorted to and whether the youth possesses a sufficiently clear idea of this virtue. Whether or not the use of the *epôdê* is necessary in this case, the requirement for the "presentation" by the patient of his soul is thus expressly and methodically fulfilled.

The result of Socrates' investigation is not conclusive. The several definitions of *sôphrosynê* which appear in succession —"doing everything in good order and with calm" (159b), "sensitivity to modesty" (160e), "each one doing what is proper for him" (161b), "practice of the good" (163e), "knowledge of oneself" (164d), "the only one of the sciences that has for its object itself and the rest" (166e), "science of knowledge and of ignorance" (169a)—do not stand up to the pressure of careful and rigorous criticism; at best, they are mere approximations of the essence of that virtue. "Here we are routed straight down the line," Socrates confesses, "and unable to describe what the lawgiver of language named *sôphrosynê*" (175b); and what is worse, we are drawn by the power of reasoning to the conclusion that *sôphrosynê* is good for nothing (175d).

What can and should be done in such a predicament? Assert that the charm of the Thracian is of no value at all? Socrates prefers to consider himself "a bad searcher" and to continue believing that *sôphrosynê* is a great good (175e). Many years later, almost at the end of his life, Plato will affirm that *sôphrosynê*, which is also present in animals and children, must be considered an irrational form of virtue (*Laws*, VI, 710a).[15] Human virtue can be irrational; learning and virtue are not in-

---

15. This does not prevent some especially talented and educated men from having an intellectual knowledge of the beautiful and the good. Such is the case of the *nomophylakes* or "guardians of the laws." In respect to the beautiful and the good these "guardians" must know "not only that which is many, but also that which is one" (*Laws*, XII, 966a). The problem of the mass and the minority thus is vigorously posed by Plato.

terchangeable terms. With this Plato, disciple and continuer of Socrates, boldly departs from Socratic thought.[16]

Charmides for his part abandons himself confidently to the procedure of his master: he believes in the goodness and usefulness of *sôphrosynê* even though his reason is incapable of proving this, and he confesses his need of it without reservation: "I am quite certain that I greatly need the charm and nothing on my part will stand in the way of my being charmed by you every day until you say that it is enough" (176b), he says to Socrates, and that decision—"to offer himself to be enchanted by him" (176b)—is for Critias, the young man's tutor, the best demonstration that *sôphrosynê* does exist in his soul.

A discussion of *sôphrosynê*, the *Charmides* is at the same time a powerful attempt to rationalize the *epôdê*. The strength of the latter, its *dynamis*, does not come to it now from any magic virtue; that strength is not a pleading, *orenda*, governable by men especially endowed therein, but something natural and inherent in the word itself, when the word is apt and beautiful. Gorgias and Antiphon had opened the way. The texts of the *Laws* in which the term *epôdê* appears will guide us to the limit of Plato's rationaling endeavor.

The figurative and not directly magical sense of the word *epôdê* is frequent in the pages of the *Laws*. To enchant with words or to charm, *epadein*, is at times, as in so many passages already cited, to make use of verbal expression with persuasive efficacy: the Athenian proposes to "enchant" Cleinias in order to convince him of something (VIII, 837e); the citing of persuasive examples is called on another occasion *epadein* (XII, 944b); with regard to the policy of marriage bonds the need to resort to the charm—that is, to the efficacious word—is proclaimed: "in order to persuade each one that he should give more importance to the equability of his children than to

---

16. At least from the radical ethical intellectualism of the Socrates to whom writers characteristically refer. The Socrates that Plato and Xenophon present to us was anything but a "pure intellectualist." See *Vida de Sócrates*, by A. Tovar (Madrid, 1947).

The Platonic Rationalization of the Charm 119

equality, never satisfied, of alliances of riches" (VI, 773d); the belief in God arises little by little through gradual persuasion of the souls of children who "have heard their nurses and their mothers sing enchanting tales, *epôdai*, at times cheerful and at times solemn" (X, 887d).

At other times every verbal device, tale, or song that serves to educate the mind of the young is called an *epôdê*. Such is the case in II, 659e; II, 665c; II, 670e; VII, 812c. The suasive effect of music no doubt increases the "enchanting" efficacy of the word; the power of the *epôdê* also springs *aus dem Geiste der Musik,* as Nietzsche would say; but the working of that which is recited or sung never fails to be decisive: "all the choruses, three in number," says the Athenian, "should enchant [*epadein*] the souls of the children while they are young and tender by saying all the beautiful things [*kala panta*] that we have already set forth" (II, 664b). The relation of these *kala panta* to the *logoi kaloi* of the *Charmides* is more than evident.

A passage from Book X enables us to become more precisely acquainted with the Platonic idea of those *kala panta*. The problem is to convince the disputants or debaters of the providence of the gods in respect to small things and of the disposition of these within the good of the whole to which they belong, and the Athenian states the advisability of adding to the discussion "enchanting myths," tales, or narratives [17] of sufficient persuasive power (X, 903b). Discussion (*dialegein*) obliges or forces (*biazesthai*) men by means of arguments or reasons (*tois logois*) to confess error and to recognize the truth; the narration of an enchanting myth, on the other hand, is able to persuade (*peithein*) the favorable acceptance (*apodechomai*) of that which can and should be believed (X, 903a).[18] This, as we have seen, is precisely the function and significance possessed by the myth of the destiny of souls in the *Phaedo*.

17. "This myth [*mythos*], this tale [*logos*], or however it need be called," it is said in IX, 872d.
18. A. Diès neatly related this opposition between the myth and the argument with the one that Plato himself establishes between the preamble of the law and the law itself, and between persuasion and necessity (*Laws,* IV, 722c).

Plato too renders tribute to the power of *Peithô*, goddess of persuasion. Myth moves the mind to receive with attention and belief that which the reason of man, or the reason of "such a" man, is not able to prove with manifest and irrefutable logical arguments.[19] With this the *epôdê* attains the pinnacle of its value.

Let us now examine as a whole the thought of Plato concerning the charm. Is his use of *epôdê* for persuasive verbal expression perhaps only a simple metaphor? Are the magic charm-*epôdê* and the persuasive word-*epôdê* wholly equivocal terms in respect to one another, with a homonymy similar to that present between "cat"-feline animal and "cat"-mechanical device to lift weights? Is the use of the same name to designate such different realities merely an ingenious vagary of the great writer Plato?

I do not think so. Plato's metaphor is, to a certain degree, a true analogy as well. The normal likening of those two realities has a firm basis in fact reducible to the two following statements: both *epôdai* are verbal expressions; both seek to produce and do in fact produce a *real and effective* change in the mind of the one upon whom they act. In the magic charm-*epôdê* there is a considerable portion of superstition and fraud, against which the philosopher and lawgiver Plato lucidly and expressly rebels (*Laws*, X, 909b; XI, 933d; *Rep.*, II, 364b); but this does not impede the hearing of it, *when it is received with belief,* from working in a real way upon the psychic, or rather indeed psychosomatic, state of the hearer. It is what we are today accustomed to call "suggestion" or "suggestive action." The beautiful speech-*epôdê* or the myth-*epôdê*, on the other hand, not only acts suggestively when the hearer is already a believer in it, but by the natural virtue of

---

19. Cf. Boyancé, pp. 155–65; L. Edelstein, "The Function of the Myth in Plato's Philosophy," *Journal of the History of Ideas, 10* (1949), 463 ff.; and J. Marías, "Introducción a Platón," *Platón. Fedro,* translated by María Araujo (Buenos Aires, 1948), pp. 93–96. As can be seen, Plato makes a very decided and express distinction between "logical evidence" and "mythical evidence"; and after having combatted Gorgias, concedes that Gorgias is partially right.

its form and content (musical modulation, character and meaning of its text) it is able persuasively to elicit a new belief in the mind of one who listens to it or to make more intense the beliefs that already existed deep within that mind. These are the common features and specific differences of the two *epôdai* and thus the true reason for the analogy between them.

In both cases—but in an outstanding way in the second, that of the beautiful speech-*epôdê* or the myth-*epôdê*—the real modification of the soul of the hearer consists in the production of *sôphrosynê*: the *Charmides* says so categorically (157a). Under the influence of the enchanting word the mind of the hearer—and subsequently his body, to the extent possible—are calmed, enlightened, and set in good order, become *sôphrones*, are "sophronized," if so expressive a neologism may be allowed. And all this in a strictly natural way by the proper virtue of that which is said, and because of the personal frame of mind of the one who hears what is said to him.[20] Plato is now a hundred leagues away from magic or sorcery in the strict sense of impious *goêteia*.

This is what I call the "rationalization of the charm." But the word "rationalization" must be taken here with a grain of salt. Plato by no means thinks that the enchanting effect of a beautiful speech or a myth is completely intelligible to the discursive reasoning of the human mind, that it is a "clear and distinct" idea, as will be said centuries later. The "rationalized" *epôdê* acts by engendering *sôphrosynê*, a virtue which, as we know, is far from being a fully rational habit for man; the beautiful speech and the myth, unlike the rational argument, work upon the mind by eliciting in it persuasive opinions and finally beliefs that are never entirely reducible to strict reason; the philosophically acceptable *epôdê* belongs in short to "the demonic," that is, to that which places men and

---

20. "The soul being of a particular nature and speeches of a particular nature [the art of oratory] teaches what is the cause by virtue of which these latter produce persuasion in one soul and unbelief in another" (*Phaedrus*, 271b).

gods in mutual relation (*Symp.*, 202e-203a). As there are false soothsayers and true soothsayers (*Charm.*, 173c), so there are false *epôdoi* and true *epôdoi*. To this second and salutary class of charmers or enchanters Socrates and Plato wish to belong when they tell their educational myths; beneath the occasional and undeniable irony of their discourse, both talk very seriously, convinced that they are aiding in a real "divinization" of the men who follow them with good will.[21] Whether *sôphrosynê* is more or less human and rational,[22] the *sôphrôn* is always a blissful man, *makarios* (*Charm.*, 175e).

The psychic health of man, a condition of his somatic health and a necessary precondition for the right administration of any medicament, consists then of the good order of the two principal parts of his soul: that in which the rational or logical, modifiable by the action of dialectic, predominates, and the other in which the irrational or the element of belief is preponderant, subject to education or *psychagôgia* (*Phaedrus*, 261a-271c) by the persuasive charm of the *epôdê*, beautiful speech, or the myth. This psychological dualism of Plato, underlying the very well-known threefold division of the soul in the *Republic* and the *Timaeus*, does not exclude the divine character of both parts of the psychic life; it could be said moreover that for Plato man is "divinely one." The *theoria*, supreme form of the exercise of intelligence, deifies man: "through living together with the divine and well-ordered," it is stated in the *Republic*, "the philosopher becomes as well-ordered and divine as a man can be" (VI, 500c-d);[23] and the same may be said, as we know, of the nonsuperstitious *epôdê*,

21. Socrates used to say, according to the testimony of Xenophon, that his friends and pupils followed him day and night to learn of him *philtra* and *epôdai* (*Mem.*, III, II, 16 s).

22. "Because of its beauty *mania* [*sc.* non-pathological *mania*] is superior to *sôphrosynê;* the former comes from God, the other is the work of men," it is stated in the *Phaedrus* (244d). It could be said that for Plato *mania* is divine by "infusion" of divinity and *sôphrosynê* by "aspiration" to it. For the social origin of *sôphrosynê*, see A. J. Festugière, *Contemplation et vie contemplative selon Platon* (Paris, 1936), p. 133.

23. It would not be difficult to gather many passages analogous to this one. On this subject see the book by A. J. Festugière mentioned above.

of poetic creation, and of all the practices and ways of living that Plato calls "demonic."²⁴ In all orders of existence, rational and faith-dominated and affective, human perfection consists of *homoiôsis theô* or the "likening of man to God" (*Theaet.*, 176a-b).

Let us now turn to the problem of the therapeutic *epôdê*. When will this *epôdê* cease to be superstitious and magical? When will it no longer be a "charm" or "conjuration" in the strict sense of these words? I believe that Plato's reply can be rightly stated as follows: An *épôde* will be philosophically acceptable and medically effective when it attains the status of a *logos kalos*, a "beautiful speech," and when the patient receives it after having first "offered," "yielded," or "presented" his soul. This poses for us the problem of knowing when the "speech" of the therapist is really and truly *kalos*, "beautiful," and what "presenting," "yielding," or offering the soul involves.

So that the word of the physician may be persuasive and may engender *sôphrosynê*, it must above all be subtly accommodated to the character and state of mind of the patient. The general precept established by the *Phaedrus* for the good orator—"to know how many aspects the soul is capable of" (271d)—cannot fail to be valid in the case of the "physician-orator"; the more so since according to the same dialogue there is a close parallel between medicine and rhetoric (27b). From the point of view of therapeutic effect, the *logos* of the physician will be *kalos* when its form and content are properly adjusted to the particular nature and situation of the patient's soul.

But we already know that the presentation, yielding, or offering of the soul is a prerequisite for the operation of the *epôdê*. No less than three times does the *Charmides* make

24. Plato is not a pure intellectualist, but he does not on that account cease to be an intellectualist. Anyone doubting this should read in *Phaedrus* of the varied hierarchy in which he ranks human souls: the philosopher and the lover of beauty occupy the first place; the seer and the participant in rites of initiation, the fifth; the poet, the sixth. In respect to the problem of the rationalism of Plato, see the chapter, "Plato and the irrational soul," in the book of Dodds previously mentioned.

this observation, and always with the same word—the verb *parechô*—as though the latter had here the quality of a technical term (157b, 157c, 176b). What, then, constitutes that *paraschesis* of the mind without which the word of the physician can achieve no effect? Plato tells us nothing; but it does not seem that Charmides could "offer" his soul to the *epôdê* (157b) or to Socrates (176b) if that act did not bring with it two things: on the one hand, the prior trusting confidence of the young man in both the efficacy of the *epôdê* with which he is to be treated and in the qualification of the physician such that the *epôdê* on his lips may be a *logos kalos,* and on the other hand in some expression of himself by means of which the therapist may become acquainted with the particular character and situation of the soul "offered" to him. When questioned by Socrates Charmides speaks of himself and of his personal opinion about *sôphrosynê,* and his behavior becomes an incipient compliance in advance with what Critias bids him do at the end of the dialogue: to yield or offer himself to Socrates to be charmed by him. Philosophical apprenticeship at Socrates' side is at once a cause of intellectual progress (157c), a source of *sôphrosynê,* and a precondition for effective therapeutic treatment.

Then what is human health? For Plato, something more than the *isonomia tôn dynameôn* or "balance of powers" of Alcmeon or the *eukrasia* or "good mixture" of the Hippocratics. In a famous passage of the *Phaedrus*—coinciding moreover with the opinion held in common by Socrates and the Thracian follower of Zamolxis in the passage of the *Charmides* commented upon above—Plato ascribes to Hippocratic medicine an excessive concern with the health of the body (270b-c). Hence he, Plato, wishes to proceed in his investigation *pros tô Hippocratei,* "beyond Hippocrates." The health of the whole man, what each man calls, without need for further explanation, "my health," is something more than a somatic *eukrasia.* It requires that the mind possess a well-ordered system of "persuasions" or "convictions" (*peithô*) and intellectual and moral "virtues" (*aretai*) (*Phaedrus,* 270b); it requires in short the *sôphrosynê* that the "beautiful speech" of Socrates must produce in the mind of Charmides. Whether or not the essence of *sôphrosynê* can be reduced to a rational definition, what is it, descriptively considered, but a set of beliefs, knowledge, appetites, and virtues beautifully and harmoniously intercombined (*kosmiôs*)? (*Charm.*, 159b). When man finds himself enjoying full and truly "human" health his *eukrasia* rests and thrives, psychologically and metaphysically speaking, in the good order of that set of psychic habits.[25] Accordingly, the disorder of the latter in some way corrupts that good mixture of humors and physical powers which make up *eukrasia* and prevents medicaments from exerting on the body all the therapeutic effect of which they are capable.[26] This is the Platonic and real meaning of the necessary temporal priority of the *epôdê* to the administration of the *pharmakon*, so expressly and insistently proclaimed by Socrates in the *Charmides*.

Note the subtlety and the profundity of the thought of Plato. When it is a matter of the *physis* of man, he tells us, in short, health, life *kata physin*, must also be life *kata peithô*, a psychosomatic activity in which the basic beliefs of generic and individual existence are in good psychological and moral order. (*Rep.*, X, 618b). Health is not indifferent to the relation of man to the Divinity, and this not only because of the fact

25. The participation of the soul as a constituent part of the state of health was asserted by Plato directly or indirectly a large number of times. I shall limit myself to referring to *Gorg.*, 526d; *Phaedo*, 89d; *Rep.*, III, 408e; *Phil.*, 63e; *Laws*, XII, 960d; *Ep.*, X, 358c. The pleasurable feeling of health and that of *sôphrosynê* (*tou sôphronein*) accompany virtue as a god is followed by his court, the beautiful passage of the *Philebus* says.

26. The usual meaning of the word "Platonic"—Platonic love, Platonic admiration—has little to do with the real Plato. To the Platonic *erôs* sexual procreation *also* belongs, that is, a strictly physical and instinctive process (*Symp.*, 206a-e). The same can be said of *sôphrosynê*, even though it is a virtue of the soul. The body is not and cannot be unrelated to it, at least before death. Without *sôphrosynê* there is no health. But can *sôphrosynê* and physical illness exist at one and the same time? Plato does not specifically take up this problem. Centuries later Christianity will give my question a decisively affirmative reply.

that Hygieia is a goddess. Therefore the rationalized *epôdê*, the *logos kalos* of the physician, is a demonic operation belonging in a special way to the relationship of man to the gods (*Symp.*, 203a); and this constitutive relationship of persuasion and belief to human health—*peithô*, persuasion, and *pistis*, belief, are words which, as we know, have the same root—is also what requires of the patient the deep and trusting confidence in the physician with which Charmides must yield or offer himself (*parechein*) to the action of the Socratic charm.[27]

Beyond the shadow of a doubt Plato thus becomes the *inventor of a rigorously technical verbal psychotherapy*. Gorgias and Antiphon are but prehistory beside Plato. Thanks to his vigorous and subtle rationalizing endeavor the old therapeutic *epôdê*, the magic charm or conjuration of ancient times, is resolved into three elements very different from one another: The magical, the rational,[28] and the beseeching. The magical element, sharply and persistently opposed by Plato, will be the only one to live on in the *epôdai* of superstitious medicine.[29] The rational element, beginning as a pure and undifferentiated suggestive action in the archaic *epôdê*, takes on the form of *logos kalos* and becomes technical psychotherapy. Technically utilized, the word acts by what it is, by the joint power of its own nature and the nature of the patient, rather than as a result of any magic power. The beseeching element, finally, will live on in the form of *euchê*, or prayer to the gods. The famous prayer of Socrates to Pan (*Phaedrus*, 279b-c) contains an implicit plea for health, and it is certain that the prayer to Helios made on the battlefield of Potideia by the philosopher must also have contained such a plea (*Symp.*, 220d).

III. These reflexions on the Platonic conception of the

27. Present-day psychoanalytical doctrines of the relationship between physician and patient are nothing but a more or less unilateral development of this Platonic *parechein*.

28. Rational, but with the exceptions that the peculiar character of Plato's rationalism demands in respect to the sense of this word. Recall what has already been said.

29. There is also some real effect of persuasive character in them. Suffice it to recall the well-known treatment of cutaneous warts by magic charms.

charm would not be complete without a study in some detail of the relation that may exist within Plato's thought between the *epôdê* and *katharsis*. Is it not true that verbal incantation and purification have been inseparably joined since the earliest times of Greek culture? "Orpheus," writes Boyancé, "is essentially an enchanter, and because he is an enchanter he is also a cathartist." [30] In a poem of Valerius Flaccus the soothsayer Mopsus sings a *carmen lustrificum* to free the Argonauts from the defilement that the murder of King Cyzicus has brought down upon them.[31] Accordingly, if the charm purifies, what is for Plato the relation existing between the *epôdê* and *katharsis*?

The Platonic idea of *katharsis* has been much studied in recent years.[32] It does not seem pertinent to take up here, even in brief summary, the content of each of such studies. It will suffice to point out, following Moulinier, that the idea of *katharsis* occupies an essential place in the very heart of Platonic thought. Hence it is that in order to solve with some degree of accuracy the problem here at issue—the relation between the therapeutic *epôdê* and *katharsis* as Plato understands them— it is necessary first to define the various senses in which the latter word is used in the writings of the philosopher.

These senses are at least five: 1. In its most neutral and workaday acceptation *katharsis* is for Plato, as for all the Greek peoples, the cleansing or purification of dirty material objects: potash serves for the *katharsis* of oil and dust stains (*Tim.*, 60d); the sieve is an instrument for the *katharsis* of grain (*Tim.*, 52e), etc. *Katharos*, "pure," is thus a body which is free of all that is not itself: pure gold, pure wine. 2. In another

30. p. 38.
31. Boyancé, "Un rite de purification dans les Argonautiques de Valérius Flaccus," *Revue des Études latines*, 1935, pp. 107–36.
32. Besides the classic *Psyche* by Rohde, and the books of Boyancé, Festugière, Dodds, and Moulinier already cited, see the article "Katharsis," by Fr. Pfister in *RE*, of Pauly-Wissowa, Suppl. Bd. 6, cols. 146–62, the inaugural dissertation of G. van der Veer *Reiniging en Reinheid bij Platon* (Utrecht, 1936), and the work of H. Flashar, "Die medizinischen Grundlagen der Lehre von der Wirkung der Dichtung in der griechischen Poetik," *Hermes, 84* (1956), 12–48.

usage, equally traditional and popular, *katharsis* is a religious concept: the purification that entry into a holy place requires, the state of purity in which certain sects place their faithful, or the ritual and punitive lustration of one who has stained himself with some crime. It will more than suffice to read as examples the frequent references in the *Laws* to cathartic rites of religious character. 3. *Katharsis* is also in several Platonic works a strictly medical concept: as in so many passages of the *Corpus Hippocraticum* the term here names the act of purging the body of the humors and impurities in it which are the cause of disease.[33] This is the meaning of the term in *Timaeus*, 72c, 83d-e, 86a and 89a-b; in the *Republic*, III, 406d; in the *Laws*, I, 628e, etc. 4. The *katharsis* which the *Phaedo* defines and advocates—that the mind purify or free itself of the body by the practice of the theoretical life [34]—is on the other hand a strictly philosophical concept. Two imperatives determined this subtle and highly refined Platonic development of the old religious and popular *katharsis:* one of religious character (to save the reality of the gods and of the "divine within us") and another of intellectual nature, at once both metaphysical and anthropological (to guarantee the reality of things, placed in question by the Sophists, and to understand what constitutes the purity of the *nous* or mind of man). 5. Finally, the word *katharsis* is used by Plato in a sense at once ethical, psychological, and medical, which it will be well to examine with special care.

Before proceeding to such an investigation it will not be out of place to point out the double bond uniting the five meanings of the Platonic *katharsis*. Firstly, among all of them there is a formal and external link, for all allude to the purity or cleansing of something. But there is also, and this is the decisive point, a deep, radical bond, firmly rooted in the very foun-

---

33. Cf., together with the cited bibliography, the monograph by W. Artelt, *Studien zur Geschichte der Begriffe "Heilmittel" und "Gift," Studien zur Geschichte der Medizin* (Leipzig, 1937).

34. Whenever we speak of "pure reason," "pure knowledge," etc., our expressions have behind them, whether we know it or not, the *katharsis* of the Platonic *Phaedo*.

dation of the reality to which each one refers: the sacred or divine character of the truly "pure," whether it be the cosmic *Physis*, the contemplation of ideas, or the psychic harmony of the man who lives according to justice. Like the reality of man under the apparent diversity of his parts and activities, *katharsis*, so varied in the writings of Plato, is also "divinely one," and this fact makes analogical, and not merely metaphorical as has sometimes been said, the use of the same word to designate things so different from each other as the washing of a piece of furniture, a lustral rite, and philosophical knowledge. Beneath the verbal and conceptual play of the metaphor there is in this case a true analogy, the analogy which the scholastics call "intrinsic."

Of the five senses indicated above the first three were current in Greece at the time of Plato, in contrast to the last two, which are wholly and originally Platonic. Plato was in fact the first to make the mind subject to "purification" or *katharsis*.[35] "The *katharsis* and the cathartic agents [*katharmoi*] of medicine and divination," says Socrates in the *Cratylus*, "all this seems to have only one virtue: to make man pure in body and soul" (405a-b). But this is the problem. What constitutes being "pure of soul"? Purity of the body is obtained by medicaments and hygienic and lustral baths. How, on the other hand, is purity of soul to be secured? And above all, what has taken place in the soul of one who has submitted himself to the *katharsis* that Plato advocates?

Let us try to collect and set in order the subtle, finely discriminating and widely scattered Platonic thoughts on the subject. The *nous*, the mind, "the divine in us"—"the pure *nous*," it is called on one occasion (*Crat.*, 396b)—is pure of itself,

---

35. The expression *kathairein tên psychên*, "to purify the soul," appears for the first time in the Socratic circle (Xenophon, Plato). It is to be supposed therefore that Socrates must have been its inventor. Until him the Greeks used the word *phrên* to say that something other than the body was impure in man. In the famous inscription of Epidaurus in which, it appears, a moral concern is expressed, *phronein* is read, and in Eleusis it was a question of *gnômen kathareuein*, "purifying thought" (Cf. Moulinier, *Le pur et l'impur*, p. 329).

hence it has no need of *katharsis*. But man is at one and the same time *nous* and living body; or, to put it more precisely, mind or *nous*, body or *sôma*, and soul or *psychê*, understanding by the latter the life of the individual body and the principle of that life. From this it is to be inferred that living man can only be *katharos*, pure, through *katharsis* of his body and his soul. "Purify the soul": this is the new watchword.[36] How is it to be accomplished?

Everyone knows the simplistic and extreme solution of the *Phaedo*. Man obtains the purity of his soul, and hence his own purity, by devoting himself to the theoretical life; that is, by acting in his life with the *nous* alone, by being pure *nous* in the measure to which this is possible in earthly existence and thus preparing himself for the bliss reserved for the true philosopher after death. The "purification of the soul," in short, consists in freeing oneself from the body insofar as possible. Sensation defiles the body and stains the soul, impregnating it with evil (65e-66b); if the soul wishes to achieve purity it must acquire the habit of "withdrawing upon itself from all the points of the body" (67c);[37] injustice, the ill of the soul, ultimately comes from the contamination by the body, and both courage (*andreia*) and moderation (*sôphrosynê*) gain their right, health-bringing sense when they are exercised in contempt of the body (68c-69a).

With this, a Platonic thought already outlined in the youthful dialogues acquires fundamental expression. Injustice and intemperance are maladies of the soul; consequently, justice is the remedy for wickedness, *iatrikê ponêrias*, Socrates says in the *Gorgias* (477b-478e). The impurity of the soul, the *Cratylus* will add, is due to the disorder of physical desires (403e-404a). Now this is so, the *Phaedo* concludes—because the body as such defiles the soul, stains it, makes it ill and needful of *katharsis*. The injustice of man must be nothing else than infection of his soul by corporality.

36. The question of whether the Orphics and the Pythagoreans spoke specifically of the *kathairein tên psychên* will not be touched on here.
37. This passage clearly indicates, Boyancé notes (pp. 83 ff), that the *psychê* is for Plato a material reality. Otherwise, I would add, the analogical character of the *nosos psychês* would not be possible (see below).

The conception of injustice and wickedness as diseases of the soul does not disappear from the subsequent work of Plato. Recall the careful definition and division of *katharsis* in the *Sophist*. Katharsis is the art of separating the good from the bad; it is in consequence *technê diakritikê*, the art of sifting or discernment. Now it seems necessary to distinguish the *katharsis* of inanimate bodies from that of living bodies, and in the latter that of the body from that of the soul. Katharsis of the body is accomplished by gymnastics, which keep away ugliness, and by medicine, which frees it from illness. Katharsis of the soul cleanses it in turn of wickedness, its most characteristic "disease" (*nosos psychês*), and of ignorance, which is but its particular way of undergoing ugliness (226c-228a). Sexual licentiousness is also a "disease of the soul" according to a passage in the *Timaeus* (86d); avarice and the scorn for gods and men were "maladies" of Achilles—of the soul of Achilles, of course (*Rep.*, III, 391c).[38]

The soul is subject to illness, from which it can free or cleanse itself by a special *katharsis*. What is the particular nature of this *katharsis*? Plato gives his reply on several occasions. But before studying the Platonic treatment of "diseases of the soul" it will be well to investigate briefly the essence, structure, and etiology of such ailments.

As in the case of the *epôdê*, a preliminary question arises to confront us. Is the express consideration of moral impurity as a disease of the soul merely a metaphorical device of Plato, or is it something more closely linked and profound? Tacitly or explicitly, recent literature seems to choose the first horn of the dilemma;[39] I am decidedly inclined toward the second. It is true that when he seeks to describe the essence and the structure of the *nosos psychês* Plato seems to limit himself to transferring to the psychic and moral order the expressions and concepts which the Hippocratic Asclepiads had developed

38. *Laws*, XI, 925e, speaks of "lacks of intelligence," *pêroseis dianoias*, in antithesis to "diseases of the body" (*sômatôn nosêmata*). Similar passages occur in *Gorg.*, 477b-c and 480b; *Rep.*, X, 609c-e and 610c; *Laws*, IX, 862c.
39. The opinion of H. Flashar is wholly explicit. For him, Plato did not go beyond using medical language metaphorically.

since Alcmeon for a scientific understanding of illness of the body.[40] The stain, or physical and moral impurity, which was somatic illness in the archaic period of Greek culture is transformed during the course of the fifth century—thanks to the rationalizing labor of the "physiological" physicians, Hippocrates among them—into *dysmetria* of the individual *physis,* into disorder and imbalance of the material elements that make up that *physis* (*dyskrasia, dysrroia*). Now this is what Plato does with moral impurity or "disease of the soul." The latter ceases to be a stain or filth, subject to being "washed away" by the material means of religious or juridical *katharsis* [41] and is converted into *ametria* of the soul, into imbalance or disorder of the beliefs, knowledge, feelings, and appetites that give the *psyché* its content and structure. As "psychological states" of a concrete man, injustice and wickedness are but morbid alterations of the good internal order of the soul, "discord" (*stasis*) of the elements that make it up (*Sophist,* 228a-d; *Rep.,* IV, 444d; *Tim.,* 87d). An unjust man must be basically nothing else than a man psychically out of tune.[42]

What are the determining causes of the disorder of which the "malady of the soul" consists? We already are acquainted with the ready and simple reply of the *Phaedo:* the moral impurity of the soul, or to use another word, its *ametria,* always comes from contamination by the body. The body: here is the enemy of the one who aspires to perfection; a human act will be more "pure" as it succeeds in being less physical and more a partaker in the free and supreme purity of the *nous.* But the mind of Plato could not remain confined within the limits of so rigid and narrow an antisomatism. The *Phaedo* had hardly been written when his doctrine began to be subtly diversified

40. See in respect to this problem my *Introducción histórica al estudio de la patología psicosomática.*

41. This does not prevent Plato—a great conservative beneath his brilliant attempt at philosophical enlightenment—from continuing to permit some of the old cathartic rites in his ideal city. Cf. the books of Dodds and Moulinier mentioned previously.

42. This does not mean that the soul is "a certain harmony," as the Pythagoreans had declared. Plato carefully makes this warning in *Phaedo,* 86c.

or revised. Gymnastics and music serve to set in order man's sensations and make them "pure" (*Rep.*, III, 411e-412a); a little later the persuasive doctrine of "pure pleasure" appears, the first example of which are the delights of the sense of smell (*Rep.*, IX, 584b-c). The *Philebus* will give substance and intellectual contour to that doctrine and will mention a whole series of "unmingled" pleasures: "those that arise from the colors that we call beautiful, from shapes and from the majority of perfumes and sounds; all the pleasures in short whose absence is not painful or perceptible, while their presence affords them to us in abundance, palpable to sense, pleasant, pure, and unalloyed with pain" (51b). For Plato, of course, there continue to be "impure" and troublesome pleasures needing *katharsis*, such as the "pleasure of scratching oneself" that he so humorously and expressively cites by way of example (*Phil.*, 51c); but his explicit and decided assertion of the existence of physical pleasures not in need of *katharsis*—fully acceptable accordingly to those who in this life aspire to perfection—plainly shows a new intellectual and affective attitude toward the reality of the body. The body as such does not defile the soul; and from the impure or "mixed" pleasures too— not even that of knowledge is unmixed, for the "hunger to know" places in it a vein of anxiety and pain (52a)—it is possible to derive something that is neither impurity nor a cause of psychic disorder and injustice.

Then what is it that places the soul in a state of *ametria*? What is the real cause of *nosos psychês*? If injustice is a disease of the soul what is the true cause of this malady? Not the body, but the disorderly act and desire: impiousness in its varied forms, crime, licentious life, the will to do mischief, and willful ignorance. All the deep, rich, religious and ethical substratum of the *Laws* is a gloss on this serene and definitive spiritual attitude of Plato. Without becoming less exacting and severe the philosopher has come to be more complex and subtle. Is not what they call "resignation" sometimes a ripening in complexity and subtlety; or, to borrow Aristotle's word (*Problem.*, 954a-b), in melancholy?

This new and finely shaded etiological conception of "disease of the soul" enables us to understand more adequately the sense in which that name was for Plato something more than a striking and convenient metaphor. In fact, between the maladies of the body and those of the soul there is not only metaphorical parallelism or *extrinsic* analogy; there is also an unbroken transition and a close genetic relationship, both in the case of diseases that we are accustomed today to call "mental" as well as in disorders of moral character, injustice, or wickedness. The former are thematically studied in *Timaeus,* 86b-87b. Plato reduces them to two types, *mania* or stark madness and *amathia* or morbid ignorance.[43] Both are etiologically related to a particular alteration of the body: "the sperm spreads and flows in waves into the marrow." But the moral "diseases" of the soul, too, can be caused by somatic diseases or be the cause of them if the body was previously healthy. "Whenever our body is unduly loosened or overstrained by diseases or other mishaps, it is a necessary result that the soul be at once destroyed" (*Phaedo,* 86c); the irritating action of a certain substance that bathes and moistens the body through the pores of the bones produces a moral disorder in the soul (*Tim.,* 86d); acting in the opposite direction immoderate desires, pains, and fears can cause man to fall ill (*Phaedo,* 83b-c). The excess of one of the parts of the soul or, in the case of injustice, the sense of guilt, the subjective discomfort that his own psychic *ametria* excites in the injust man, is able to produce somatic disorders—if you will, psychosomatic—of a strictly morbid character. Put in other words: without *sôphrosynê* complete physical health is not possible.[44]

At this point we can understand with full clarity the Pla-

---

43. The debate of H. Flashar (pp. 23-24) with A. E. Taylor (*A Commentary on Plato's "Timaeus",* Oxford, 1928) in regard to this page of the *Timaeus* could in my opinion be solved by taking into account that in this dialogue Plato is speaking of strictly medical or psychiatric diseases of the soul, while the *nosos psychês* of the *Sophist* has reference rather to moral disorders, wickedness (*ponêria*), or culpable ignorance (*agnoia*). The *amathia* of the *Timaeus* would correspond approximately to what we today are accustomed to call "mental retardation."

44. Through another route there appears here a notion already revealed on previous pages.

tonic *katharsis* of the "diseases of the soul." What can the *katharmoi* be, those cathartic agents able to restore order in souls affected by *ametria*? Perhaps the fumigations with sulfur or the lustral baths of traditional *katharsis*? Only in the measure in which such practices exert a suasive and educative effect upon the soul of one who undergoes them, [45] for it is wholly evident that the proper *katharsis* for moral disorder can be no other than the suitable and suasive word, the *epôdê*, in the most Platonic sense of the term. From time immemorial the Greeks had been using song and recitation for specifically cathartic purposes. Plato accordingly, remaining within that old tradition but rationalizing it religiously and philosophically, terms *katharsis tês psychês,* "purification of the soul," the proper verbal reordering of the beliefs, knowledge, feelings, and appetites that give content to the "soul" of man; *dia tou logou katharsis,* "purification by the word," a neo-Platonist will say centuries later.[46]

There are not a few passages in which Plato alludes expressly to that verbal and rationalizing *katharsis* of the "diseases of the soul." A line of the *Cratylus* declares priests and Sophists to be experts in purificatory operations (396e); here Sophism, the art of persuading through the word, is conceived of as verbal *katharsis*: the profession of the good Sophist is to "purify" the souls of those who hear him in their need. The ingenious etymological fantasies on the name of Apollo in that same dialogue have an analogous meaning. Apollo is the god of divination and medicine.[47] Both purify the body and the soul, the body by means of baths, sprinklings, and medicaments, the soul by means of the true word of the oracle of Delphi. Socrates concludes that Apollo, faithful to his name, is a god who washes (*apolouôn*) and unties (*apolyôn*) and at the same time is truthful (*talêthes*) and without guile, sincere (*haploun*) (405b). The Pythia, through

45. Recall what has been said in respect to the "conservative" character of Plato. Against the Greek *polis* Plato proposes to save what Dodds calls the "Inherited Conglomerate."
46. Eunapius, *vit. soph.* 474s. (ed. of Fr. Boissonade).
47 And also of music and of the art of the bow (*Crat.*, 405a).

whose mouth the god of Delphi speaks, works a true divinatory and medicinal *katharsis* with the truth of her word.[48] No less clear is the allusion to the true verbal *katharsis* of the "disease of the soul"—in this case, injustice against the gods—in the *Phaedrus* where Socrates decides to follow the example of Stesichorus [49] and "wash" with the sweet water of a speech the bitter salinity of the offenses inflicted upon the god of love (243a-d). The recantation thus has a decisive cathartic effect.[50] But the dialogue in which "purification by the word" is most roundly and specifically affirmed is the *Sophist* (229d-230d). We already know that the *katharsis* of the soul must free the latter of wickedness and ignorance if in fact one or the other makes it ill. What can the agent of that purification be? How will an unbalanced soul, disordered by *ametria*, be able to recover the sound and beautiful composure of moral health? By means of punitive correction and the educative word, is the concise reply of Plato. But the latter comprises at one and the same time two different arts, the art of persuasively admonishing and that of arguing or refuting effectively.[51] The two manners of action of the word which Book X of the *Laws* distinguishes, the compulsive or dialectical manner and the suasive or mythical, emerge under a new guise in these subtle discriminations of the *Sophist*.

There is no doubt: for Plato, the cathartic agent that the "malady of the soul" specifically requires is the apt and effective word. By imparting convincing proofs or by instilling persuasion, the verbal expression of one who knows how to be at

48. The same in *Phaedrus*, 244a-e. The truth cleans and heals: this is the essence of Platonic thought about verbal *katharsis*.

49. According to the legend, Stesichorus went blind from having insulted Helen in his poem, "The destruction of Troy." To recover his sight he had to "purify" his soul by means of a specific retraction. "Palinôdia" was the title of this new poem.

50. The *katharsis* by the word is in this case *ex ore* and not *ex auditu*. Elsewhere (*Estudios de Historia de la Medicina y de Antropología médica*, Madrid, 1943) I have set forth at some length the theory of these two modes of verbal *katharsis*.

51. It cannot be surprising, according to this, that Plato should call the *elegxis* or convincing argument "the highest and principal one of the *katharseis*" (230d).

one and the same time teacher and physician—"psychagogue," Plato would say—is able to reorder souls affected by *ametria* and restore them to their true essence. "No man is voluntarily bad," the *Timaeus* teaches (86d). The essence of man is naturally *emmetron*, well proportioned, and hence the process of purifying him of what he is not proves curative. This appears to be precisely the effect that the *katharsis* "by the word" produces in the soul of those who undergo it.

The essential connection between *katharsis* and the *epôdê* is now outlined with complete clarity. Every *epôdê* is a verbal *katharmos*, a means for the purification of the soul by means of the word. The *epôdê* engenders *sôphrosynê;* and the latter, whatever its ultimate essence may be, manifests itself descriptively as a well-regulated and lucid composure of all that which makes up the soul of man: beliefs, knowledge, feelings, and impulses. More than temperance or moderation derived from contempt for the body, as the extreme puritanism of the *Phaedo* could maintain, *sôphrosynê* is *kosmos*, "good order and control of the pleasures and appetites," so that "that which by nature is best may prevail over that which is worst" (*Rep.*, IV, 430e-431a). And is not the serene possession of this *emmetria* or well-ordered proportion of the soul (*Rep.*, VI, 486d) perhaps the end to which verbal *katharsis* should lead, as Plato understood it? It cannot be surprising that the Platonist Chion, or the writer who later took that name, asserts that philosophy is *epôdê*, beneficent charm (*Ep.*, 3, 6 p., 196 H). Such had been the innermost nerve of the intellectual and ethical teaching of his master.

IV. Let us now view in retrospect our investigation as a whole. A careful examination of the Platonic conception of the charm has thrown some light on three different fields, the history of medical knowledge, general anthropology, and the theory of verbal expression.

The preceding pages oblige us to see Plato as the inventor of scientific, or *kata technên*, verbal psychotherapy. Beside him, as already remarked, Gorgias and Antiphon are mere prehistory. The philosopher never forgot his discovery in the

Charmides. At the very end of his life, reflecting intermittently upon what the physician should do, he will write: "The free physician—the one who does not attend to slaves—shares his impressions with the patient and the latter's friends; while he informs himself about the patient at the same time insofar as possible he instructs him and prescribes nothing without having persuaded him beforehand, and thus, with the aid of persuasion [*meta peithous*], soothes and continually disposes him so as to lead him little by little to health" (*Laws*, IV, 720d-e). Without the psychagogic work of verbal persuasion the therapeutic work accomplished by medicaments, diet, and surgical incision would not be entirely effective nor totally human—would not be appropriate for "free" patients and physicians. The imperative of the rationalized *epôdê*, an imperative so subtly discovered in that youthful dialogue, continues to maintain its full vigor in the writings of extreme old age.

In respect to general anthropology, the Platonic meditation on *epôdê* and *katharsis* enables us to understand from a favorable point of view the relation between that which in man's being is rational, subject to manifest logical intellection, and those ingredients of the human reality which today we are accustomed to call irrational. The famous "intellectualism" of Plato can thus be more correctly understood.

Finally, the Greek doctrine of the psychological and ethical effect of the word becomes more clear and articulate. The considerations of Aristotle on the persuasive effect of the rhetorical syllogism, or syllogism of probability (*enthymêma*), and the debated sentence of the *Poetics* in which the Stagirite mentions the cathartic process of tragedy doubtlessly take on a fresh prominence when they are examined from the point of view of this victorious intellectual battle by Plato against the magic of the *epôdê* and *katharsis*. But before studying the Aristotelian doctrine of the tragic catharsis of the passions, we shall do well to examine with some care the attitude of the actual physicians—the followers of Asclepius who composed the *Corpus Hippocraticum*—toward the problem of therapy by the word.

Chapter 4

The Word in Hippocratic Medicine

More or less foreseen by the poets and the first philosophers, later outlined by the Sophists and developed by Plato, a doctrine of the therapeutic use of the human word was established in Greece between the second half of the sixth century and the first half of the fourth century B.C. Now this is the period of Greek history in which "technical," "physiological," or "scientific" medicine is born and grows: the science and art of healing of the physicians later called "Hippocratic." Alcmeon of Crotona—"young when Pythagoras was old," according to Aristotle (*Met.*, 986a)—must have composed the works from which his famous and decisive fragmentary passages are derived around the year 500 B.C. A little later the physician Herodicus of Selimbria, the probable teacher of Hippocrates, practiced with general renown. Thirty years older than Plato, Hippocrates, born, as is well known, about 460, could read the works of Gorgias and Antiphon and not a few of the dialogues of the great Athenian philosopher as well. It is a well-substantiated tradition that Hippocrates was a pupil of Gorgias and Democritus. Moreover a good portion of the writings of the *Corpus Hippocraticum* was composed in the fourth century, and it is almost certain that some of them come from a still later period.[1] It can therefore be asked: What did the authors of the *Corpus Hippocraticum* think and what did they say

1. Edelstein assures us ("Hippokrates," *R.E.*, Suppl. Bd. 6, col. 1331) that the writings of the *Corpus Hippocraticum*, despite their different dates and sources, come from the fifth and fourth centuries; he indicates as an exception only the seventh book of the *Epidemics*, composed, according to Herzog (*Abh. Akad. Berl.*, 1928, 6, 38), in the third century. But more recently U. Fischer ("Untersuchungen zu den pseudohippokratischen Schriften *parangeliai peri iêtrou* und *peri euschêmosynês,*" *Neue Deutsche Forsch.* Berlin, 1939) thinks on good grounds that *peri*

about therapy by the word? What was the reception accorded to that which the Sophists and philosophers thought and said on this subject?

In the following pages I shall try to give a satisfactory answer to these questions. But I must not begin my task without clearly setting forth the method that I am going to follow and the reasons that justify it. The variety of the writings that make up the *Hippocratic Collection* is without doubt extraordinary. To the divergencies for which the different dates of the several works are responsible must be added those that result from their varied subject matter (theoretical, medical, surgical, gynecological, etc.) and those that reflect the particular intellectual orientation of each author, either because of the school to which he belongs or as a result of his personal peculiarity.[2] Thus it occurs that the various writings not only differ from one another but even debate among themselves in not a few cases. However, this undeniable fact having been openly recognized, I give advance notice that in my study I shall consider the *Corpus Hippocraticum* as a unified whole. When required, I shall accord the necessary attention to the special meaning given a passage by the work to which it belongs; but this will not stand in the way of its organic connection with the other passages. Two reasons justify this method:

---

iêtrou is a product of the third century and that two other works were composed during the second period of Sophism (first to second centuries A.D.). Jaeger, for his part (*Paideia,* 3, 53) believes that *peri diaitês* was written "well into the fourth century."

2. My references to the Hippocratic bibliography—so copious a bibliography since Littré and the *Hippokratische Untersuchungen* of C. Fredrich (Berlin, 1899) and yet still so insufficient—will always have a selective character. In respect to that internal diversity of the *Corpus Hippocraticum,* see the works of Edelstein, Schumacher, Nestle, and Jaeger already cited, and in addition: L. Edelstein, "*Peri aerôn*" *und die Sammlung der hippokratischen Schriften* (Berlin, 1931), and "The Genuine Works of Hippocrates," *Bull. of the History of Medicine,* 7, (1939), 136–48; K. Deichgräber, *Die Epidemien und das Corpus Hippocraticum,* Abh. Preuss. Akad. der Wiss., 1933; H. Diller, *Wanderarzt und Aitiologe, Philologus,* Suppl. Bd. 26, 1934; W. Nestle, "Hippocratica," *Griechische Studien* (Stuttgart, 1948). The Hippocratic texts will always be given with reference to the edition by Littré (L.), the volume and page being indicated with Arabic numbers.

1. Despite the differences that in fact exist among the various writings of the *Hippocratic Collection,* and with the exception of those few later than the fourth century, the aggregate of these writings is what made up as doctrine the *technê iatrikê* of the Greeks during the "golden age" of Hellenic medicine and what therefore determined the course of the history of Western medical knowledge ever since. In an investigation of the importance of the therapeutic word in Greek medicine a unified view of the *Corpus Hippocraticum* is a necessity.

2. The so often mentioned internal diversity does not rule out the existence of a basic and deep-seated unity among the various treatises that make up the *Corpus.* Something fundamental causes the disagreeing authors to coincide and to resemble one another, something because of which both the pneumatic work *On the Winds* and the humoral work *On the Nature of Man* are to our eyes, and certainly to the eyes of a Greek physician of the fourth century, "Hippocratic medicine." The possibility that Temkin opened up years ago with his search for a "systematic correlation" (*systematischer Zusammenhang*) deep within the *Corpus* has not in my judgment been sufficiently utilized.[3] It is necessary to make precise and careful distinctions; otherwise there would be no science. But it is also a good thing, according to the familiar saying, for the trees to let the forest be seen, and the *Hippocratic Collection,* despite the considerable number of different trees that make it up, is a venerable forest.

Let us now take up our subject; let us endeavor to determine what reality and significance the word had in Hippocratic medicine. "Word" in Greek is *logos.* Now what was the *logos* and what did it mean in the thought and practice of the Hippocratic physicians? In order to solve this historical problem we must not forget that the term *logos* had two main senses among several others—"reason" and "word"—and in addition that the human word can be expressive and communicative. In consequence let us begin by studying what the *logos,*

3. O. Temkin, "Der systematische Zusammenhang im Corpus Hippocraticum," *Kyklos, 1* (1928), 9–43.

as reason and expressive word, was in Hippocratic medicine.

I. That by means of which man can "give an account" of reality and express in his mind or with words what is rational or at least reasonable in things received from the Greeks the name of *logos;* which is the same as to say that the *logos* is the highest means of intellectual knowledge. If the mind or *nous* of man is able to know reality it is because he has *logos,* because man is by nature an animal endowed with *logos: logon echon,* "possessor of *logos,*" Aristotle will later say. If reality in turn can be known by man it is because the cosmos has deep within it an immanent reason or order, a sovereign *logos.* Such was the brilliant discovery of Heraclitus that Empedocles, Anaxagoras, and Democritus subsequently inherited and put to use. And since Hippocratic medicine became established as a science in the lap of pre-Socratic *physiologia,* could that double-headed idea of the *logos* not have been active in the intelligence of its creators: the *logos* as reason—the reason of man, the reason of the being of things—and as the expressive word?

I need not set forth here the little that is known about the gradual development of "scientific" medicine during the archaic age of the Greek people.[4] I shall limit myself to recalling once more the Pythagorean ancestry of Alcmeon of Crotona and to stating that in the evolution of this "scientific" or "physiological" medicine—not to speak of the fundamental thing: the intellectual and technical maturity of the Greek genius in the fifth century—three different historical processes join together: one empirical (the accumulation of experience by the nomadic and stationary practitioners able to do so),[5] a second of religious character (the medical cult of Asclepius

4. The book by Ch. Daremberg, *La médecine entre Homère et Hippocrate* (Paris, 1869), is still valid for the most part. See also R. Fuchs, "Geschichte der Heilkunde bei den Griechen," *Handbuch der Geschichte der Medizin,* ed. by Neuburger-Pagel; W. Nestle, *Vom Mythos zum Logos;* and J. Schumacher, *Antike Medizin.*

5. A funerary inscription of the sixth century makes known to us the existence of an eminent physician named Charon in Titronius of Phocis (Nestle, *Vom Mythos,* p. 208). There must have been many others like him, whose names we do not even know.

had something to do with Hippocratic medicine),[6] and a third of philosophical nature (pre-Socratic thought about the *Physis*). This last was doubtlessly the fundamental and configurative process. "Why," Jaeger asks himself, "did a medicine as developed as that of Egypt never become a science, as we think of it? The Egyptian physicians certainly did not suffer from a lack of specialization, already very pronounced among them, nor from a lack of experience." And Jaeger replies: "The solution of the riddle cannot be more simple: it consists purely and simply of the fact that those men did not adopt toward nature as a whole the philosophical point of view that the Ionians were able to adopt . . . The Greek physicians, disciplined by the thought of their philosophical predecessors, were the first able to create a theoretical system that could serve as basis for a scientific movement."[7]

The detailed and systematic explanation of what may be considered in Hippocratic medicine as "fundamental and general doctrine" also goes beyond the limits of my present aim. Again I must refer the reader to the manuals of the history of medicine and the monographs previously mentioned. But it would not be possible to show the meaning of the word in Hippocratic medicine without noting briefly and synoptically the principal innovations that the latter offers in respect to what we might rather freely call the "medical thought" of archaic Greece. The five are, in my opinion, the following:

1. From the point of view of its "essence" disease ceases to be something superadded in a disturbing way to the individual reality of the patient (*lyma, miasma,* or *daimôn*) and is conceived of as an internal "disorder" of that reality. The idea of that disorder, prefaced by the notion of *monarchia* ("predominance of one of the powers") that Alcmeon of Crotona had brilliantly introduced, will be expressed in Hippocratic medicine in the form of *ametria* (disorder of the powers), *dyskrasia* (disorder in the mixture of the humors), or *dysrroia*

---

6. I refer the reader to the works of Edelstein and Herzog already cited.
7. *Paideia,* 3, 14.

(disorder in the flow of the pneuma). The "physical stain" is thus changed into a "disharmony of the *physis*."

2. From the point of view of its "cause" disease ceases to be the result of possession, defilement, or punishment and is seen as the effect of a "natural" process sufficiently anomalous and violent to upset in a pathological manner the double dynamic equilibrium—inner equilibrium of the body, equilibrium between the body and the cosmos—of which health consists. Disease is now "punishment" only when the violation of the good order of Nature has been the fault of the patient; in another case disease is *atychia*, a chance misfortune, incomprehensible and free of guilt. "There are no diseases that are more divine than others," the works *On Airs, Waters and Places* and *On The Sacred Disease* agree.

3. Therapeutic practice consequently ceases to be routine empiricism, a magical process or the "purification" of the patient, and is changed into an "art" or *technê*, into *technê iatrikê*. Medicine is the first of the *technai* within the little differentiated traditional "learning" to acquire its own reality both intellectually and socially, hence its unquestioned prestige in Greek life of the second half of the fifth century and the exemplary quality that the medical art often acquires in the minds of Sophists and philosophers, whether they be called Socrates, Plato, or Aristotle.

Technê for the Greeks was a knowing how to do, made up of two essentially interdependent capacities of the man—the "artist" or *technitês*—who possesses it: knowing *what is* that which is being done (what the ability put into practice "is") and worked on (what the reality to which the "art" is applied "is"), and knowing why one does what is done when one acts "according to art." "Art" displaces "magic" forever. The *technitês* of medicine must know what treatment and diagnosis are, what man is, what disease is, and what the remedy is; with all these he will know satisfactorily why he does in each case what correct treatment requires. Moreover, by making the *technê* a means to knowledge he will even come to believe that "only through medicine will it be possible to learn something certain about [human] nature" (*de prisca med.*, 20, Littré *1*, 620–22).

4. All this demands the possession of a satisfactory idea of the *Physis*. Could medical knowledge of the "nature" of man and of the "nature" of the remedy be attained without a prior and fundamental scientific knowledge of "nature" in general, without *physiologia*? The pre-Socratic *physiologia* was thus the *arché* or "principle" of Hippocratic medicine in the two main senses that the word *arché* had for the Greeks: the sense of "beginning" (chronological principle) and that of "foundation" (constituent principle).

What was *physis* for the Hippocratic physicians? [8] Fundamentally, the "nature" of the totality of all things and the "nature" of each thing in particular; or as Book I of the *Epidemics* says, the *koiné physis apantôn* or "common nature of all things" and the *idié physis ekastou* or "proper nature of each thing" (L. 2, 670); if you will, *Physis* and the *physeis*.

In its most general definition *physis* is not the mere sum of all the "natural things" that exist, but what is fundamental and primary in the totality of them all, something that for a Greek was at one and the same time unitary, procreative, harmonious, and divine. The Hippocratic physician was no exception to this rule. In the *Corpus Hippocraticum* the reality of *physis* is unitary; everything has *physis:* [9] "all diseases have *physis* and none originates without it," says the author of *On Airs, Waters and Places* (L. 2, 78). It is also fecund, life-engendering: the work *On the Nature of the Child* (*Peri physeôs paidiou*) is not so much about the anatomical and physiological constitution of the infant as about its origin, and thus one understands that these pages are a continuation of the brief treatise *On Procrea-*

8. The problem has been philosophically studied by Nestle, Diller, and Deichgräber. Their respective works have been mentioned on previous pages.

9. The *nomos* is not *physis*, but assumes it. See Diller, *Wanderarzt und Aitiologe*, p. 57. The *nomos-physis* antithesis has two versions in the *Corpus Hippocraticum:* one pre-Sophistic (contrast between Europeans and Asians in *On Airs, Waters and Places*) and another Sophistic: "In this respect—it is stated in *On Diet*, I—usage (*nomos*) is opposition to nature (*physis*)" (L. 6, 476).

tion. The verb *phyein* meant, as we know, to grow or germinate. *Physis* is also harmony, not only static or resultant harmony but also the cause of harmony, an active and efficacious principle of order. What is in good morphological and functional order is "according to *physis*," *kata physin.* The passages of the *Corpus Hippocraticum* in which the teleology of *physis* is asserted are well known: "Natures are the physicians of diseases. Nature finds the ways by herself, not by reflection . . . Well instructed by herself [*eupaideutos*],[10] without a learning process, she does what is best" (*Epid.*, VI, L. 5, 314); "Nature suffices herself in all for all . . . Natures do not have a teacher in anything" (*De alim.*, 15 and 39; L. 9, 102 and 112). It was not without consequence that the word *kosmos*, from which "cosmology" and "cosmetics" are derived, meant in Greek "universe" and "embellishment" or "adornment." The reality of *physis* is, in short, divine. Neither the religiosity of the Hippocratic physician (*de morbo sacro*, L. 6, 358) nor many passages of the *Corpus* could be understood without taking that divine character of *physis* into account. When we are told in *On the Sacred Disease* and in *On Airs, Waters and Places* that epilepsy and the effeminacy of the Scythians are maladies no more "divine" than others (*de morbo sacro*, L. 6, 364 and 386; *de aere, aquis et locis*, L. 2, 76), because all diseases are "equally divine and human" (L. 6, 394) and "none is more divine nor more human than the others" (L. 2, 76), what is meant is that the diseases of man are "natural" accidents and that all have divine—and of course human—character in whatever pertains to their existence as "natural" processes; in short, that *physis* is universally divine (L. 6, 364). The natural course of things is accomplished "with divine necessity" (*ananké theié*), one reads in *On Diet* (L. 6, 478); thus if *physis* is opposed to the efforts of art, all is useless (*Lex*, L. 4, 638). The first lines of the work *On Virgins* have in my judgment a like sense: "The principle [*arché*] of medicine is the constitution of lasting things [*aieigeneôn*, eternally generated and eternally generating]" (L. 8, 466). What sense, ac-

10. I follow Jaeger's reading (*Paideia*, 3, 45), as opposed to *apaideutos*, "without instruction," that Littré adopted.

cording to this, can the passing allusion to "the divine" in the *Prognosis* and in *On the Nature of Woman* have? In the former work it is stated that the physician "must discern whether there is something divine [*ti theion*] in diseases" (L. 2, 112); in the latter one reads: "Here is what I say about the nature of woman and her ailments: the divine is the principal cause in human beings; then come the natures of women and their colors" (L. 7, 312). That is to say the physician must be aware of whether there is something "naturally" insuperable in diseases, of whether the "divine necessity" of *physis* is at work in a perceptible way in their appearance and their course. That which is "natural"—hence "divine"—in men is the basic thing in their reality, and afterwards come the typical and individual sexual qualities which color at times expresses. Centuries later at the height of Hellenism the author of *On Propriety* will explain that the good physician in the face of spontaneous or "natural" cures feels moved to revere the gods (L. 9, 234). *Physis* beyond doubt was for the Hippocratic the divine, *to theion*.[11]

Physis is manifested and realized in the *physeis*, the particular "natures" of specific things. In other words, in what each thing has of its own or "by nature" in the totality of its natural properties. This restricted definition of the word *physis* will allow the Hippocratics to speak of the *"physis* of man" (L. 6, 32) or even more specifically, of the *"physis* of the backbone" (*de artic.*, 45, L. 4, 190). The anatomy, embryology, and physiology of the *Corpus Hippocraticum* with its various "dynamic," humoral, or pneumatic explanations were but the expression of a scientific knowledge about the particular *physis* of man as a part and product of the general and universal *physis*.

5. This technical knowledge and language concerning *Physis* was called *physio-logia;* it was accordingly the *logos* of the human *physis* in a state of health and illness. Hippocratic

11. In addition to the publications mentioned—especially the work of W. Nestle, "Der Begriff des *theion* und *daimonion*," *Griechische Studien* —see H. W. Miller, "The Concept of the Divine in *De Morbo Sacro*," *Transactions and Proceedings of the American Philological Association, 84* (1953), 1–16.

medicine, so considered, was the result of a particular employment of the *logos,* the latter being understood both as the reason of man and things and as expressive word. The fifth of the great innovations that shine out in Hippocratic medicine was the formation of a *logos iatrikos* or "medical reason." Let us try to fathom its structure.

The cognitive *logos* of the Hippocratic physician had the *physis* of man—more specifically, in the somatic aspect of that *physis*—as its subject and object: object, inasmuch as the *physis* is in itself "reasonable," as Heraclitus had taught; subject as well, inasmuch as it is the "natural reason" of man which keeps awake and proclaims that inner rationality of the *physis.* The author of *On Places in Man* asserts this very clearly: "The *physis* of the body is the principle [*archê*] of the *logos* in medicine" (L. 6, 278). That is, the nature of the human body is the reality to which the *logos* of the physician is above all to be applied. He who does so will discover that the *physis* is regular in itself: that "for those who know [human nature] it is always straight-forward or regular [*aiei orthôs*] and for those who do not know it, always irregular [*aiei allôs*] in one way or another," according to the compact formula of Book I of *On Diet* (L. 6, 488). Therefore the wise physician who knows divine nature and aids it to win back lost order when it is ill is, so reads a famous sentence, "like a god": *iêtros gar philosophos isotheos* (*de hab. dec.,* 5, L. 9, 232).

The conviction that Nature is in itself regular and reasonable may enable one to understand concordantly the sense of a considerable number of antitheses scattered through the writings of the *Corpus Hippocraticum. Logos* and *ergon,* word and work, appear sometimes in opposition (*Praecepta,* 2, L. 9, 252) and on other occasions in a complementary relationship (*de vulner. cap.,* 10, L. 3, 214); in the first case when the *logos* of the physician departs from the reality of the *physis,* in the second when it adheres faithfully to it. "Eyes, not words," asks the brief treatise on the reduction of dislocations (*Vect.,* 36, L. 4, 381); that is, eyes faithful to the *logos* of the *physis,* not misguided and vain speeches, *logoi*. Therefore experienced men know the value of the right word and are more content to prove by works (*ergôn*) than by speeches (*logôn*) (*de arte*, 13, L. 6, 26); and for this reason too the wise man should prefer his intelligence to his eyes if he is trying to know what things are under the mantle of their immediate appearance: "It is an opinion of people that what grows from Hades into the light is born, and what diminishes from the light to Hades dies. More trust is placed in the eyes than in the intelligence [*gnômê*] when they are not sufficient even to discern what they see. For my part, I ask explanation of the intelligence" (*de diaeta*, I, 5, L. 6, 474). The author of the discussion *On the Art* contrasts to the conventionality of the names of things imposed upon Nature by the judgment of man (*nomothetêmata*) the spontaneous and emergent reality of the "aspects" of the former (*eidea*): these must be "productions" or "formations" (*blastêmata*) of Nature and in their contemplation the well-oriented intelligence should seek nourishment (L. 6, 4).[12] "There are two things—*The Law* teaches in accordance with the Eleatic philosophers—science [*epistême*] and opinion [*doxa*]; the former creates knowledge, the latter ignorance" (L. 4, 642). The first is the work of the right and true *logos;* the other, a product of the fleeting and superficial *logos*.

The concrete employment of the *logos* as reason is "reasoning" or *logismos;* and since there is a *logos iatrikos*—the *logos* that enables what health and disease really "are" to be known —there must be also a "medical reasoning." This reasoning

12. The medical, philological, and physiological questions that the use of the terms *eidea, idea,* and *eidê* in the *Corpus Hippocraticum* poses are important. In my study on Hippocratic clinical history (*La historia clínica*, Madrid, 1950, pp. 29–64) I saw in them the first outline of the "morbid species" of traditional pathology. Jaeger, for his part (*Paideia*, 3, 33, 36, and 54), supported in the works of A. E. Taylor (*Varia Socratica*, Oxford, 1911) and G. Else ("The Terminology of the Ideas," *Harvard Studies in Classical Philology*, 1936), writes: "When a typical variety is distinguished, one speaks in medicine of *eidê*, but when it is simply a matter of unity within variety, the concept of *one idea, mia idea*, is used instead." The logos of the physician discerns the "ideas" of reality.

can be diagnostic or therapeutic. "When the physician has not been able to determine the malady by direct visual observation nor by information heard, he searches it out by reasoning," the author of *On the Art* (L. 6, 20) tells us. Reasoning becomes especially necessary when the morbid change is inaccessible to the sight, and it adopts at times in practice the form of a true "test under stress' or "functional test": "Thus medicine at one time forces the innate heat to dissipate out the phlegm by tart foods and drinks in order to support its judgment by the sight of something in cases in which it would otherwise be absolutely impossible to discern anything, at another by means of walks uphill and running obliges the *pneuma* to reveal that of which it is a revealer" (*de arte*, 12, L. 6, 24). But the physician will never reason without taking into account the results of his sensory observation. "Reasoning," the *Praecepta* warn in a cautious and Aristotelian manner, "is a sort of synthetic memory of what has been gathered by the senses" (L. 9, 25). Here is the subtle pattern that Book VI of the *Epidemics* proposes for the proper guidance of a diagnostic judgment: "Make a summary of the origin and onset [of the disease] and of many meditations and detailed examinations, scrutinize the concordances [of the symptoms] among themselves, and then the discordances among the concordances, and finally new concordances among the discordances, until a single concordance is derived from the discordances: this is the way" (L. 5, 298). By this mental process the physician comes to know the inner order of the symptoms and understands their apparent diversity from a central point of reference; which would be impossible if such reasoning (*logismos*) did not rest directly upon a scientific doctrine (*logos*) in respect to the human *physis*.

But the therapeutic process also demands that reason be put into practice in the course of reasoning. "The same reasoning [*logismô*] can lead one to take [in the treatment] opposite routes," one of the *Aphorisms* teaches (*Aphor.*, IV, 9, L. 4, 504); "medicine has reasons [*logous*] at its disposal that afford it means for the treatment," the author of *On the Art* emphasizes (L. 6, 26). But this will occur only when the reasoning is reasonable in itself, when it rightly obeys the *logos*. This is how the curious opposition between *logismos* and *logos* contained in this precept must be understood: "To practice medicine one must not follow the first persuasive reason [*tribê meta logou*]" (*Praecepta*, 1, L. 9, 250–52). Along with reasonings faithful to the *logos* of the *physis* there is always, as a danger, the possibility of others merely probable or fallacious, based rather on opinion than on truth. But when it is the former that the intelligence uses, the *logos* of the physician has the propriety and the force of a "just law" (*nomos dikaios*) (*de fract.*, 7, L. 3, 442). Stirring in truth and good, the *nomos* is just and at harmony with the *physis*. Hippocratic thought is thus much nearer to Democritus than to Antiphon.

II. In the *Corpus Hippocraticum* the *logos* is primarily reason and expressive word; but it is also—and this now pertains directly to our theme—a communicative word, a telling others, in short, a question, reply, or speech in the rhetorical sense of this latter term.[13] The Hippocratic physician, besides expressing with his *logos* what reality "is"—the fraction of reality that is of concern to him as a physician—speaks to communicate with someone: the gods, the patient, or the persons around him. Let us continue and consider in order each of these diverse forms of the communicative word.

The word addressed to the gods technically receives the name of "prayer," *euchê*. The Hippocratic physicians were not unaware of it; at least those whose views find expression in Book IV of the work *On Diet*. "Thus, after having determined the celestial signs," it is stated with respect to dreams in which torments appear, "the physician will take precautions, will follow the indicated regimen and will raise prayers to the gods" (L. 6, 652). The beseeching intention is now evident; the physician asks the gods—the context indicates very precisely

13. In my books *Estudios de Historia de la Medicina y Antropología médica* (Madrid, 1941) and *La empresa de ser hombre* (Madrid, 1958), can be read a description of the psychological action of the word that considerably enlarges upon that proposed by Karl Bühler in his *Psychologie der Sprache*.

which ones—for the result of his prescriptions to be favorable. But can one who, like the Hippocratic physician, believes in the "necessity of nature" and in the divine character of that necessity appeal to prayer with the ingenuous confidence of the man who is not a *physiologus?* The author of the fourth book of *On Diet,* debating with the interpreters of dreams who apply the same criteria to "physical" dreams, or those caused by the body, as to "divine" dreams, or those sent by the gods, says: "They are content to prescribe prayers. Praying is doubtlessly a proper and good thing; but even when invoking the gods it is necessary to help oneself" (L. 6, 642). In other words the physician has to reckon on the insufficiency of his art, but he should endeavor primarily to insure that his prescriptions are in harmony with the divine necessity of nature. Such is the thought implicit in the work *On Places in Man* when its author methodically contrasts fortune (*tychê*) and science (*epistêmê*): "Fortune is sovereign, it does not obey orders and even prayer does not fetch it; but science obeys and brings good fortune when he who possesses it wishes to make use of it" (L. 6, 342). The best prayer of the physician, according to this, would be to act piously and technically, in accordance with the divine necessity of the *physis.*

More frequently than to the gods the word of the Hippocratic physician was addressed to the patient and to those around the patient. But the intent of the speaker was not always the same. At least five different intents—and accordingly at least five types of communicative medical word—may be distinguished in the *Corpus Hippocraticum.* In its pages the medical word is in fact question, prescription, instrument of prestige, means of enlightenment, and persuasive agent.

The communicative speech of the physician becomes "question" or "inquiry" (*ereuna, erôtêsis*) and *anamnêsis* (recollecting, calling to mind). The most varied writings in the *Corpus Hippocraticum,* some of general character, others at the service of a very concrete and determined purpose, point out the need to question the patient if the physician would act according to art. "Questioning the patient and examining everything with care . . ." says the author of *On Diet in Acute Diseases* (L. 2, 436). A concise note in Book IV of the *Epidemics* directs the attention of the physician toward "what and how the patient himself explains; how to receive his explanation, the speeches" (L. 5, 290). And similar statements are made in *On the Diseases of Women* (L. 2, 114), in *On Wounds of the Head* (L. 3, 214 and 240), and in so many other passages of the *Hippocratic Collection*.

In the medical history the physician's question is necessary but the patient's reply is not sufficient. This should not surprise us. The patient does not speak of himself in accordance with science but according to his opinion; according to his "feeling," in the fullest sense of this word. "In the information that individuals subject to hidden maladies try to give to the physician, they speak more from opinion [*doxazontes*] than from knowledge" (*de arte*, 11, L. 6, 20). Hence the type of knowledge that questioning offers the physician is not science but conjecture: "Whoever in regard to treatment would interrogate correctly, answer the questions and rightly reply," it is stated in *On Diseases*, "must recall . . . what is done or is said by conjecture [*eikasiê*] by the physician to the patient or by the patient to the physician" (L. 6, 140). Diagnostic and therapeutic judgments based on the words of the patient are conjectural. Dependence upon them alone is not therefore the behavior of experts but an error of the ignorant. The method of the authors of the Cnidian maxims must have been such as this. "They have proceeded," it is said in *On Diet in Acute Diseases*, "like one ignorant of medicine: he would be able to give an accurate description of diseases by carefully gathering information from patients about what they are experiencing" (L. 2, 224). The physician must know what the patient cannot tell (*ibid.*) and investigate accordingly "what can be perceived by looking, touching, listening and by smelling, tasting, and understanding" (*de offic. med.*, 1, L. 3, 272). Was it not indeed rigorously necessary, according to the diagnostic pattern of the *Epidemics*, carefully to taste the earwax?

The word of the Hippocratic physician is in other cases a

"prescription," a means to inform the patient of what he must do in the treatment of his disease (*ta prospheromena: Epid.*, I, L. 2, 670); or a "precept" suitable to the instruction of the medical student (*dogma: Lex*, 3, L. 4, 640; *parangelia*, L. 9 250). This character of the communicative word does not require special comment.

But the case in which the word of the physician expresses a prognostic judgment does. The prognosis or prediction (*prognostikon, prognôsis, prorrêtikon, prolegein*) belongs essentially to the *technê* of the Hippocratic practitioner. If the course of the natural processes obeys an inner "necessity" (*anankê physeôs, theia anankê*), a physician will never be able to say that he knows the *physis* of a patient unless he can announce what will happen to that *physis* in the future. "It is necessary to tell the prior conditions, to know the present state, to predict the future," the *Epidemics* teaches (L. 2, 634). In the case of patients who do not feel their malady, "it is up to the physician to predict what is threatening them," warns the work *On the Joints* (L. 4, 100). So considered, prognosis constitutes an essential part of the diagnosis.

But the prognostic *logos* is not only an expression of knowledge, it is also a means of prestige both to obtain the trust of the patient and to shine socially in the city. "It seems to me that the best physician is," the *Prognosis* begins by saying, "the one who knows how to know in advance. By fathoming and explaining in advance in the presence of patients the present, past and future of their ailments, by describing what they omit, he will gain their trust [*pisteuoite*]; convinced of his superiority they will not hesitate to submit to his care. And he will also treat diseases the better when he knows by means of the present state how to predict the future" (L. 2, 110). Proceeding thus the physician "will be justly admired" (L. 2, 112), especially if the patient is intelligent (*Prorret.*, 2, L. 9, 10). The adjectives used in the *Corpus Hippocraticum* in high praise of accurate predictions well show the importance attributed to the prestige that such predictions confer. They are called indeed beautiful (*kalai*), admirable or wonderful (*thaumastai*), brilliant (*lampra*), spectacular (*agonistika*) (*Prorret.*, 1, L. 9, 6; *de artic.*, 58, L. 4, 252). But this prestige can only be admissible if the prediction is "scientific" and is based on a correct knowledge of the nature of the patient: "Brilliant and spectacular predictions," says the text of *On the Joints*, "are derived from diagnosis that foresees in what way, in what manner and in what period of time each malady will end, whether its course is toward recovery or whether toward incurability" (L. 4, 252). This is the only way not to commit an error common among bad physicians: the error of "not promising to cure the curable and promising to cure the incurable" (*de morbis*, I, 6, L. 6, 150).[14]

Let us now take up the fourth type of communicative word, that in which the word is a means of enlightenment. In the Hippocratic period the social situation of Greek medicine found itself subject to a powerful ambivalence. It was on the one hand the knowledge of a community of men religiously and technically initiated into the secrets of disease and healing, hence a knowledge forbidden to laymen. "Holy things," says *The Law*, "are revealed only to holy men; it is forbidden to impart them to laymen until they have been initiated into the mysteries of the science" (L. 4, 642). "I shall impart the precepts, the oral lessons and the rest of the instruction to my children, to the children of my master and to pupils bound by a pledge and an oath according to the medical law, but to no other," prescribes the *Oath* (L. 4, 630). But on the other hand, as Jaeger has so convincingly demonstrated, Greek medicine

14. The hunger for prestige and fame was very intense in the soul of the Greek physician; with it he manifested his Hellenic character and the persistence of the *shame culture* within the *guilt culture*. Even in the Hellenistic period the *Praecepta* will say: "At times you will lend your services gratuitously, bearing in mind the memory of an obligation or the present reason for your reputation" (L. 9, 258). The text continues, prescribing to the physician that he aid ill and poor foreigners, "for where the love of man [*philanthrôpiê*] is, the love of the art [*philotechniê*] is also." *Philanthrôpia* was one of the moral motivations of the Hellenistic physician; the culture of the period so demanded. The real sense of this connection between the "love of man" and the "love of the art" cannot be discussed here.

was from the fifth century an important part of the education or *paideia* of the private individual, of the *idiotês*, even though he was not going to devote himself to the art of healing. The author of *On Ancient Medicine* points out the need to write medical doctrine in a way intelligible to the average citizen (*dêmotês*) (L. *1*, 572); the treatise *On Affections* for its part asserts the advisability of the layman, the mere "private man" or *idiotês*, acquiring a certain amount of medical education (L. 6, 208). Thus it can be understood that a part of the writings in the *Corpus Hippocraticum* are pleas on behalf of the art of healing (*On the Art, On Breaths, On Ancient Medicine*) or explanations addressed simultaneously to the technical training of the physician and to the scientific education of the cultured man (*On the Nature of Man, On Healthful Diet, On the Sacred Disease, On Diet*). In all these cases the word of the physician taught the layman.[15]

The enlightening or clarifying intention of the *logos iatrikos* is more strictly medical when it is addressed to the patient himself for the purpose of explaining his disease. Read the page of the *Laws* in which Plato contrasts the practice of the physician of slaves and the behavior of the physician of free men. The former goes running from one patient to another and gives his prescriptions in a routine way without reasoning them out (*aneu logou*). And Plato continues: "If one of these should hear a free physician speaking with free patients in terms very similar to those of scientific lectures, explaining how he understands the disease in its origin and going back to the nature of all bodies, he would surely burst out laughing and would say what the majority of so-called physicians retort at once in such cases: What you are doing, you fool, is not curing your patient but teaching him, as though your mission were not to return him to health but almost to make a physician out of him" (*Laws*, 857c–d). That such enlightenment of

---

15. The physician's purpose was at times polemic and even defamatory. The author of *On the Art* reproaches physicians who with "words that are not beautiful" (*logôn ou kalôn*) slander other physicians, without contributing anything new of themselves (L. 6, 2).

the patient was a relatively frequent practice in Plato's day cannot be doubted; that such a procedure had considerable therapeutic—psychotherapeutic—importance in the view of the philosopher, is made clearly evident in another paragraph of the *Laws*, already cited in the previous chapter (*Laws*, 720d–e). Does this mean that the Hippocratics saw in this practice an essential part of medical treatment according to the art? This does not appear very well established. According to passages in the *Corpus Hippocraticum*—quite rare in this connection—the explanation by the physician to the patient aimed to achieve the confidence of the latter, the prestige of the former, or the factual substantiation of knowledge that the Asclepiad previously possessed. As for the winning of confidence and prestige, recall what has been said above. And as for the role of the explanation as proof, note what the author of *On Ancient Medicine* states:

> The speeches and the inquiries of a physician have no object other than the maladies of which any man falls ill and suffers. No doubt those ignorant of medicine cannot know in the case of their own diseases how they begin and end, nor why they wax and wane; but if these things are explained by those who have discovered them they will find it easy to become acquainted with them; because then they need merely to recall, as they listen to the physician, what they themselves have experienced. If the physician does not succeed in making himself understood by laymen and does not place his hearers in this state of mind, he will not attain [knowledge] of what things are. (L. *1*, 572–74)

That is to say, the harmony between the knowledge of the physician and the thinking that the patient carries out for himself when his mind is guided by the word of the other is a criterion of truth; which indicates that this word now has a much more noetic than therapeutic purpose. Hence only when it makes the patient confident of the capacity of the physician, only then may the enlightening explanation have a vague and relative psychotherapeutic significance.

Must we conclude from this that the Hippocratics were ignorant of the use of the persuasive word? Was the therapy of the word as the Sophists and Plato had understood it an idea absolutely foreign to the mentality of the authors of the *Corpus Hippocraticum*? This fifth type of *logos iatrikos*—the word as a means of persuasion and a therapeutic agent—must be the object of a more detailed investigation.

III. The principal types of the therapeutic word are, as we know, two: the magic charm and persuasive or suggestive speech, the *epôdê* and the *logos pithanos*. The Hippocratic physicians are acquainted with the *epôdê*; it could not be otherwise, since they are Greeks and men of their time; but their attitude toward the magic charm, the attitude of a "technician" educated in the pre-Socratic idea of the *physis* and of knowledge, is of frank and even violent rejection. On three occasions "agents of purification and charms" (*epaoidai*) are named in *On the Sacred Disease*, always to be impugned with obvious vigor, with abuse of the wizards, cathartists, charlatans, and imposters who use them as treatment for epilepsy (L. 6, 354, 356, and 362). Epilepsy is no more divine than other diseases; all are equally divine and equally human; Divinity, the highest purity, cannot defile man, the frailest being of Nature; to attempt to gain power over the gods by means of charms is the worst of blasphemies. In short, the medical *epaoidê* can be nothing but superstition or imposture. The diatribe against the soothsayers who deceive certain ill—perhaps hysterical, to judge by what is said of them—women, by having them consecrate clothing and objects of value to Artemis, has the same meaning (*de virgin.*, 1, L. 8, 468). It is highly probable that those soothsayers too used *epôdai* in their supposed cures.

May that vigorous rejection of the magic *epôdê* be accompanied, as in the Platonic dialogues, by a reasonable evaluation of the suggestive word and of its efficacy as a therapeutic agent? The *Corpus Hippocraticum* knows the importance that the person of the patient and of the physician possess for the effectiveness of the treatment. "It is necessary for the patient to help the physician to combat the disease," says Book I of the *Epidemics* (L. 2, 636); "It is necessary," the *Aphorisms* emphasize, "not only for one himself to do what he should, but also for the patient, the helpers and external circumstances to contribute to it" (L. 4, 458). But of what shall this active cooperation of the patient in his treatment consist? First of all firmly to trust the ability of the physician attending him. This requires that the technical knowledge of the therapist be real and at the same time his personality be able to make this evident with dignity and tact. "He who prescribes . . . can give rise to fears and hopes," the author of Book I of the *Epidemics* says also (L. 2, 670). Two of the latest works of the *Corpus*—*On the Physician* and *On Decorum*—paint a very complete portrait of the ideal physician. The physician should be a man of healthy color and not too thin of body, because not a few persons think that a man who cannot cure himself cannot well cure others; he will dress with dignity and neatness and he will perfume himself discretely, "for all this pleases patients"; he will be upright and temperate in his life, grave and humane (*philanthrôpon*) in his manner; without going so far as to be jocular and without failing to be just, he will avoid excessive austerity; he will always remain in control of himself. "So should the physician be tempered in mind and body" (*de medico*, 1, L. 9, 204–06). Much more detailed and concrete are the prescriptions of the brief treatise *On Decorum*. The physician and the sage must be "dignified without affectation, austere in their encounters, ever ready to make rejoinder, hard to contradict, perspicacious and communicative in matters agreed on, moderate toward all, silent in time of trouble, resolute and firm to silence, well prepared to seize an opportunity; . . . and they will speak asserting with their discourse insofar as may be possible everything that has been shown, making use of eloquence . . . and corroborated by the good reputation that issues from it" (L. 9, 288). Entering the room of the patient, the physician shall "remember the way to take his seat, his self-possession, his dress, grave demeanor, brevity of speech, unshakable serenity, diligence in the patient's presence, care, response to objections" (L. 9, 238–40); and he will proceed in all "with calm, with skill, concealing from the patient while he is at work most things, encouraging him [*parakeleuonta*] with cheerfulness and serenity . . . and now admonishing him with vigor and severity, now consoling him [*paramytheesthai*] with care and good will" (L. 9, 242).

In these paragraphs there is the description of a verbal psychotheraphy of unspecific character; designed accordingly to win the trust of the patient and to keep his psychosomatic tone—in everyday terms, the "good morale" of his spirit—at a good level as a prior condition for the efficacy of the treatment. It is true that these instructions come from a work which may well have been composed as late as the first century A.D.; but nothing prevents us from supposing—recall the vivid portrayal by Plato in the *Laws*—that this way of practicing medicine was usual several centuries earlier. A brief note from the sixth book of the *Epidemics* and a prescription of the second book of the same treatise show that the importance of a general or basic psychotherapy had been discovered long before the author of *On Decorum* lived. The note in question alludes to "indulgences" (*charites*) to patients and says as follows: "Cleanliness in their drinks, in their food and in everything that is offered to their view; softness in what is in contact with their body; allow whatever is not of harmful effect and is easily amended, for example, cold water when it is necessary to make this concession; visits, words, appearance, dress . . . long hair, nails, scents" (L. 5, 308). The prescription for its part refers to the re-establishment "of good color and the good distribution of the humors" and bids "the movements of the spirit, happiness, fears and other like feelings be stimulated; if this state is involved with a disease of the rest of the body, it shall be treated; if not, this is sufficient" (L. 5, 126). As is evident, it is a question here of producing a certain somatic effect by means of a kind of psychoaffective exercise. Clearer is the appeal to the somatic effect of pure suggestion in a crafty and most unscientific formula to be found in Book VI of the *Epidemics:* "If there is an earache, roll wool around the finger, pour on a little of some hot oily substance and then, having placed the wool in the palm of the hand, place the hand under the ear so that the patient may think that this will do him some good"; and the formula ends by saying with comic and nonchalant sincerity: "deceit (*apatê*)" (L. 5, 318).

All this warrants the formulation of three provisional conclusions: 1. The Hippocratic physician was not unaware of the importance of a general or basic psychotherapy in the treatment of patients. 2. The Hippocratic physician knew the somatic efficacy of the psychic life and how to use it therapeutically. 3. The Hippocratic physician knew how to use the suggestive word as a psychotherapeutic agent.

The mention of the soul is in fact not very frequent in the writings of the *Corpus Hippocraticum*, and it does not appear an accident that in the treatise *On Diet*—composed well in the fourth century and very probably influenced by the Babylonian East, Orphism, and the Platonic Academy, as Palm and Jaeger suggest—the use of the word *psychê* turns out to be most abundant.[16] "The soul of man and the body like the soul have their good arrangement [*diakosmeetai*]," says Book I of *On Diet* (L. 6, 478); and in the care of that dual "good arrangement" the good physician has his principal duty. But neither is it unusual for the other writings of the *Corpus* to refer to a psychosomatic correlation and to describe its medically important aspects. "Bodies as well as souls differ widely and have great power," the *Prorrheticus* warns (L. 9, 34); the emaciation of the soul, like that of the body, can be the cause of humoral apostasis, the treatise *On the Humors* teaches (L. 5, 488); "if the soul is burned up [*ekpyrôthê*] by illness, it consumes the body," the fourth book of the *Epidemics* asserts (L. 5, 314), based probably, like the treatise *On Diet*, on the con-

16. Palm, *Studien der Hippocratischen Schriften;* Jaeger, *Paideia,* 3, 56–57. See also W. Müri, *Bemerkungen zur hippokratischen Psychologie,* in *Festschrift für E. Tièche* (Bern, 1947). The identification of the soul with fire is very clear throughout the entire work *On Diet*. I shall limit myself to referring the reader to L. 6, 486, 514–16, 574, and 576. The influence of sounds upon the soul—to cite but one typical example—is thought of as a problem of heat and dryness (L. 6, 574–76).

ception of the soul as fire. The human soul, which is thought (*gnômê*) and hence consciousness (*xynnoia*)—it is stated in another passage—"by itself, without organs and without material things, grieves, rejoices, is frightened, takes cheer, hopes, scorns; as in the case of the portress of Hippothous, who with her thought (*gnômê*) alone learned the circumstances of her malady" (*Epid.*, VI, 8, 10; L. 5, 348). The Orphic idea of the soul, a soul capable of "separate" action, seems to be behind that view of psychic activity.[17]

Knowledge of the psychic life of man must be all the more important for the physician inasmuch as there exists a certain correlation between the character of the passions and the part of the body in which they are located and upon which they act. Here are two highly significant passages: "Anger [*oxythymiê*] contracts the heart and the lungs upon themselves and summons to the head the heat and fluids while a good frame of mind [*euthymiê*] expands the heart . . . Exercise is food for the limbs and the flesh and sleep for the viscera. For man thought is a perambulation of the soul" (*Epid.*, VI, 5; L. 5, 316). The psychosomatic correlation cannot be more vigorously and elegantly expressed. The second passage says:

> As to the soul excesses in food and drink, in sleeping and waking, and those resulting from certain passions as, for example, the game of dice, and from prolonged work either in the practice of the professions or from necessity, and in one's labors regularity or irregularity and changes, and in the latter vicissitudes. And as to the moral habits [*ek tôn etheôn*], the toilsomeness of the soul, seeking, busying itself, looking, speaking, and from other like

17. The idea of a "separate" activity of the soul must have been quite general in Greece during the first half of the fifth century. Aristotle believed in it when he was young, in the period in which he composed the *Eudemus* and to which the reports of Proclus (*In Rempubl.*, II, 1211, 1.22 ff) and Cicero (*De divin.*, I, 25, 53) refer. Aristotle, according to Proclus and Clearchus, tells of having seen how a magician was able "to separate" the soul from the body. It must have been a trick of hypnotism.

manners such as worries, fits of passion, desires; everything that accidentally troubles the thought, either through the eyes or through the ear. How then the body behaves: the scraping of a millstone sets the teeth on edge; the legs of one who walks on the edge of a precipice become weak; the hands tremble when a very heavy burden has been lifted; the sudden appearance of a serpent makes one turn pale. Fears, modesty, afflictions, pleasure, wrath and other emotions; so the part of the body corresponding to each one of them obeys each in these cases, sweats, palpitations of the heart and other phenomena due to such faculties. (*de humor.*, 9, L. 5, 488-90).

The psychic life alters the body in a selective manner. Hence words can do so too, for "things heard are beneficial or distressing" (*Epid.*, VI, 8, 7; L. 5, 346). This is no doubt the understanding of the author of Book IV of *On Diet* when he asserts that the sight of wandering stars in dreams is a sign of "disturbance of the soul because of some care [*hypo merimnês*]," and he prescribes to the patient that he "address his mind to theatrical performances, especially those that bring laughter; or otherwise to those that please him most" (L. 6, 648-50).

The reading of the latter paragraphs—in which all or almost all that approaches present-day "psychosomatic medicine" in the *Corpus Hippocraticum* has been set forth in order—may cause it to be thought that psychotherapy had a clear significance and an important place in the minds and practice of Greek physicians of the fourth century. Nothing could be farther from the truth. As I have said repeatedly, the Hippocratic texts of psychotherapeutic character aim at excessively general, unspecific goals: winning the confidence of the patient and keeping the tone of his spirit at a good level. The physician of ancient Greece did not go beyond this. Gorgias and Antiphon had begun an orderly and etiological consideration of afflictive states—their "species" (*eidê*), their "occasion" (*kai-*

ros), and their "cause" (*aitia*)—as the basis for a "technical" and effective treatment of the pathological affliction. A little later, at a date surely prior to many of the Hippocratic writings, Plato developed the whole of a brilliant doctrine of the psychic and somatic action of the word, hence of verbal psychotherapy. It is certain that a practical and consistent cultivation of the Platonic viewpoints would have soon led to the construction of something like a "Greek psychotherapy." Now, not even the slightest trace of all this can be discovered in the *Hippocratic Collection*. This fact proves all the more strange if one thinks of the almost certain student-teacher relationship between Hippocrates and Gorgias, and especially if one takes into account the close structural and genetic connection that existed between Hippocratic medicine and the art of rhetoric. Explained with crystal clarity by Plato (*Gorg.*, 464b, 465a, 501a; *Phaedrus*, 270a–d), that connection must already have been glimpsed and commented upon in the Socratic circle. Hippocrates, says Plato, teaches us to inquire always and above all whether the nature of the object upon which our *technê* is to be exercised is simple or multiple; if it is simple, it is necessary to investigate how or in what measure it is able to influence another specific object or undergo the influence of the latter; if, on the contrary, it is multiple, it will be necessary to enumerate and describe its various forms and to find out in respect to each one of them what we should have to know if it were a matter of a simple object, asking ourselves how it influences others and how it may be influenced by them. This would not be possible unless one endeavored to understand the nature of the object in question—the body in the case of medicine, the soul in the case of rhetoric—from a knowledge of "the nature of the whole" [*tou holou physeôs*] (*Phaedrus*, 270c).[18] As medicine proceeds in its intelligent effort to be a *technê*, Plato concludes, so should rhetoric proceed. But

18. On this parallelism between the Hippocratic method and the rhetorical method, see the works of Edelstein, Deichgräber, Nestle, and Jaeger previously mentioned. Whether that *holon* or "whole" to which Plato refers is the "whole body" as Edelstein declares, or the "whole universe" as Deichgräber holds, is a question that cannot be discussed here.

which art was the first to do so, medicine or rhetoric? Had not Gorgias indeed, the probable teacher of Hippocrates, discovered for himself the need that the rhetorician has to speak according to the *eidê* and the *kairos* of the minds of those who listen to him? To judge by the information given by Plato himself, rhetorical thought and medical thought must have interlaced and influenced each other more than once during the second half of the fifth century and the first decades of the fourth. Therefore the almost total silence of the *Corpus Hippocraticum* on the therapeutic action of the word is all the more surprising, as is the extraordinary practical and theoretical vagueness of its writings in everything having to do with psychotherapy.

I shall attempt to demonstrate the thesis that I am now discussing—the paucity and the vagueness of Hippocratic psychotherapy—by two series of documentary arguments, the first relative to the psychic preparation of the patient for the medical treatment, and the second concerning the therapeutic behavior of the Hippocratic Asclepiad in the case of psychosomatic diseases and conditions as much needful of suggestive cure as of the prescription of medicaments; or, as the Socrates of the *Charmides* would say, in as great need of *logos kalos* as of *pharmakon*.

Gorgias used to boast of the rhetorical skill with which he would persuade his brother's patients to accept the latter's treatments. The *Corpus Hippocraticum* for its part establishes the need for the patient to collaborate in some way in the therapeutic task of the Asclepiad. But what do the writings of the *Corpus* tell us about the concrete procedure of the physician? In the opinion of the author of *On the Art*, failure of the patient to follow therapeutic advice is more probable than error on the physician's part in prescribing it. And considering the gravest and most extreme possibility, that of a fatal end of the illness, he defends his opinion thus:

> The physician performs his duty sound of mind and sound of body, reasoning in respect to the present case and among those past ones that are similar to the pres-

ent, to the point of being able to cite cures due to the treatment he is employing. But the patient, who does not know his disease, nor its causes, nor in what his present state will end, nor what occurs in cases like his, receives the advice suffering in the present, frightened of the future, full of his ailment, empty of food, more desirous of that which his malady makes pleasant for him than of that which is best for his cure, doubtlessly not wishing to die but incapable also of resisting with determination. Which of these two events is more likely: that a patient so disposed will fail to carry out or will carry out badly the advice of the physician, or that the latter, working under the conditions described, will err in his advice? Is it not more probable that the one will prescribe what he should and that the other, incapable no doubt of being persuaded and hence unpersuaded [*mê peithomenous*] will cast himself away to death? (L. 6, 10–12)

A careful reading of this passage, so skillfully rhetorical in itself, well shows that the practice of persuasion was not very usual among the Hippocratics and arouses serious doubts as to the persuasive capacity of their words. In the presence of the patient—in the presence of patients as well disposed to the work of suggestion as those here portrayed—the Hippocratic Asclepiad did not wish or did not know how to be a "rhetorician" in the sense of Gorgias, Antiphon, and Plato. As to the acceptance of advice, the persuasive power of the physician, the use of "persuasive reasoning" or *logismos pithanos* that the *Praecepta* (L. 9, 250–52) and *On Decorum* so plainly scorn, must have been less potent than the particular nature of the patient and hence less decisive than it. "It is necessary to bear in mind," says the *Prorrheticus*, "the character of the intelligence and the physical strength of patients, because some obey easily or with difficulty one piece of advice, and others another" (L. 9, 14–16). The *physis* of the patient, then, with his particular character and his free will, decides rather than the *nomos* that the enlightening and suggestive word of the physician tries to establish.[19] As I have already noted, the verbal explanations of the physician in the presence of the patient accomplished for the Hippocratic a function more cognitive than therapeutic.

A detailed analysis of the Hippocratic procedure as respects patients in whose case psychotherapeutical treatment seems to us today most indicated brings us to the same conclusion. Here are two cases among many possible examples, one of hypochondria and one of female hysteria. The first appears in the work, *On Diseases:* "Worry, a difficult ailment: the patient seems to himself to have in his entrails a thorn that is pricking him; anxiety torments him; he flees from the light and from men; he likes darkness; he is prey to terror; his diaphragm seems to protrude and is painful if it is touched; he is afraid; he suffers from frightful visions and terrible dreams; he sees the dead. The malady usually comes on in spring" (L. 7, 108–10). The second comes from the treatise *On the Nature of Women:* "If the womb goes toward the liver, the woman immediately loses her voice, clenches her teeth, and her color grows dark. These accidents affect her suddenly and in full health. They arise particularly among old maids and among widows who, being still young and having had children, continue in widowhood" (L. 7, 314). What does the treatment of these two cases consist of? To the hypochondriac is prescribed hellebore, purging of the head and belly, donkey's milk, limitation of food and exercise, cold diet; to the hysterical woman, manual pressure upon the belly below the liver, a bandage about the spleen, pouring perfumed wine in the patient's

19. In this same sense the prudent prognostic proviso that appears on more than one occasion in *On Fractures* should be interpreted: "The cure is complete at the end of some forty days if the patients remain in bed" (L. 3, 452); "The cure takes place in sixty days if the patient remains quiet" (L. 3, 458). Gorgias would not have spoken this way. I repeat what I have said before: in his relationship to the patient, the Ascelpiad did not wish nor know how to be a rhetorician; in the acceptance of his treatments, nature and the freedom of the patient had more weight than the suggestive power of the therapist, which—from another point of view—does not speak against the Hippocratic physician.

mouth, fetid fumigation of the nose and aromatic fumigation of the womb, purges, donkey's milk, and pessaries with various vegetable preparations.[20] Of like character is the therapy prescribed in the work *On Diet* for the treatment of dreams whose content runs counter to the acts and thoughts of the day before (emetics and morning walks: L. 6, 642–44), and the inexpensive prescription against "anxiety" (*alyké*) that Book II of the *Epidemics* suggests (taking wine mixed with an equal portion of water: L. 5, 136) is the product of analogous mentality.

In all these clinical and therapeutic descriptions the predominantly psychic state of the symptomatic picture is quite obvious. Now, the Hippocratic, for whom, as we know, the great influence of the soul on the health and sickness of man was no secret, neither applies his vigorous etiological mentality to the investigation of the possible psychic reason for the disturbance nor hits upon the idea of utilizing a psychic, psychotherapeutical treatment in order to restore the unsettled psychic order. It might be said that in these cases the soul of the patient does not exist for the physician and that the classification of the curative arts that Plato proposes by way of tactics in the *Phaedrus* (medicine, the art of curing the disorders of the body; rhetoric, the art of setting straight the disturbances of the soul) had established itself in the view of the Asclepiad as a canon not to be touched. In Books V and VII of the *Epidemics* the neurosis of a certain Nicanor is succinctly described: "Whenever he would engage in drinking, the fluteplayer would frighten him; whenever he heard the first sounds of a flute at a banquet, terror seized him; he used to say that he could hardly contain himself, if it was at night; but if he heard that instrument in the daytime he was not upset. This condition of his lasted for some time" (L. 5, 250 and 444). In the face of this picture, the etiological and psychotherapeutic indifference of its depictor could not be more complete. We would

---

20. The work *On the Diseases of Women* (L. 8) describes several cases similar to this latter, both in the symptomatic picture as well as in respect to the treatment.

say that he could not be more olympic if the divine therapists Apollo and Paeon had not dwelt on Olympus. What the author of Book I of *On Diet* teaches is true: that "the soul can be made better or worse by regimen [food, baths, exercise]" (L. 6, 522). But as much as *diaita* itself—or, if you will, skillfully included in it—is not the persuasive and exemplary word man's best device to bring it about that a soul is made better?

Giving now a definitive character to the conclusions set down previously in a provisional way, we must now say: the Hippocratic could have been and even began to be a psycotherapist, but he did not do it adequately. Why? Two reasons seem to me decisive. One is accidental and tactical: the rejection of the magic *epôdê* in the name of physiological medicine. The justified and laudable vehemence with which the author of *On the Sacred Disease* argues against the charmers by superstition or by imposture may have prevented him from noting what the poets and the Sophists of the fifth century had already discovered: that there are nonmagical "verbal incantations" able to modify the reality of one who listens to them and subject accordingly to being utilized as therapeutic agents. It is not pure chance that the *Corpus Hippocraticum* is unaware of the metaphoric or analogical use of the term *epôdê*.

But another reason, no longer tactical and accidental but formal and substantive, has greater importance than this: the irrepressible tendency of the Hippocratic to see and understand the twofold nature of man somatically and indeed *only* somatically. Medicine needs a *metron,* a measure to verify the accurateness of its observations, it is stated in *On Ancient Medicine:* "now, that *metron* with reference to which the exact truth may be known is not a weight nor a number, but the sensation of the body, *tou sômatos aisthêsis*" (L. *1,* 588–90).[21] The tardy opinion of the *Praecepta,* on the other

---

21. For the signification that the measure-weight-number series had in Greece of the second half of the fifth century and the first half of the fourth, see A. J. Festugière, *Hippocrate. L'Ancienne Médecine* (Paris, 1948), pp. 41–43.

hand, should be recalled: "Reasoning is a sort of synthetic memory of what sensation has gathered" (L. 9, 250). For five centuries the perception of the body through the senses was a permanent canon of Hippocratic medicine, alpha and omega of the *technê iatrikê* as Hippocrates understood it and taught it to be understood. A great and immense achievement. Thanks to it Western medicine was able to be a science and to begin its glorious history with discipline and fecundity. But may not its loyalty to that valuable formal principle have been at times excessive? May it not have occasionally led, in respect to the reality of man, to misidentifying *physis* and *sôma* and consequently to scorning all knowledge about the human *physis* that cannot rapidly and conveniently be reduced to "sensation of the body"? The incapacity of Western medicine for verbal psychotherapy until a few decades ago depended ultimately on that great achievement and that great limitation of Hippocratic medicine.

Let us return to the lesson of the *Phaedrus*. Socrates, after having invoked the example of Hippocrates to build the art of rhetoric, asserts the need to proceed in that task "beyond or above Hippocrates," *pros tô Hippokratei*. Here is what Western medicine did not know how to do up to the end of the nineteenth century: to act at one and the same time "from Hippocrates," *pros tou Hippokratous*, and "beyond Hippocrates," *pros tô Hippokratei*. That was the only way to be rightfully and wholly faithful to man's reality, in which the state that we are accustomed to call "illness" is *always* body, but is never *only* body—the arduous and complex way that the Hippocratics were intelligent enough to glimpse but not to see and follow with sufficient clarity and decision.

Chapter 5

The Power of the Word In Aristotle

The most important part of the medical legacy of Plato—his personal view of verbal psychotherapy—was not taken up by the followers of Hippocrates in the second half of the fourth century. Undoubtedly they were ignorant of it.[1] Will Aristotle, the greatest heir and greatest contradictor of his master, succeed in doing so? Intellectual tradition is established by those who know how to inherit and know how to contradict as well; or, if you prefer, by those who know how to contradict and know also how to inherit. The philosopher of Stagira belonged in the fullest sense to this race of men. Let us repeat then the foregoing question: did Aristotle take up that medical legacy of Plato? The reply must be twofold; it must be: yes and no. No, because the work of Aristotle, the fraction of Aristotle's work that has come down to us, nowhere alludes to verbal psychotherapy, unless it be to mention in passing the practice of magic charms.[2] Yes, at the same time, because Aristotle carries Platonic thought concerning the operation of the word to the highest precision, and because medical lore is a principal resource in this intellectual undertaking of the Stagirite.

Plato had taught that the communicative *logos* can adopt two distinct forms and produce, consequently, two different psychological effects. There is on the one hand the dialectical *logos*, which by means of convincing reasoning forces the

---

1. The singular position of Diocles of Carystus in respect to the *epôdê* will be commented upon in the final pages of this book.
2. Perhaps there may have been something in the lost works. It is indeed strange that a subject so constant in Plato was not discussed or commented upon by Aristotle. There are allusions to *epôdai* of magic character in the *Historia animalium*, VIII, 24, 605a (revelant to the diseases of horses) and in fragment 454 (the conjuration to transfer a plague to crows, which I have already mentioned on previous pages).

truth to be known and recognized; in contrast stands the mythical *logos,* able to elicit belief through persuasion and to lead to a determined acceptance of what it says. The latter may be a forerunner of the former when the truth to be known is accessible to human reason, and its follower when the truth being sought is not rationally accessible to the one seeking it: "Genesis is in respect to essence what belief is in respect to truth," Plato says on one occasion (*Tim.,* 29c). Belief may be the human way to possess truths that can be known and that have not yet come to be known.

Accordingly a considerable part of the work of Aristotle is the result of a brilliant and systematic development of that Platonic distinction. The several writings that make up the *Organon*—"Categories," "Analyses," "Topics," "On Interpretation," "On Sophistic Refutations"—are but a treatise on the dialectical *logos.* The practice of the latter now receives the technical name of "logic"; its principal form is the strictly defined "syllogism" or "logical syllogism"; its purpose, the convincing and the conviction of the hearer; its subject matter, the necessary or convincing truth, the truth that inexorably imposes itself upon the intelligence. A well-constructed logical syllogism leaves one who hears it convinced and convicted, whatever his personal individual character may be; conversely, every conviction of rational character, even though it has not been obtained discursively, can be expressed by a logical syllogism or by a series of them. But as a pupil of Plato Aristotle well knows that the human word can persuade as well as convince. Together with the dialectical *logos* there is as its complement a rhetorical *logos,* the *logos* that the art of rhetoric teaches us to utilize. Hence there will be also a "rhetorical syllogism," the "enthymeme," whose name by itself (*en* and *thymos,* "in the spirit") already indicates that its psychological operation is more "cordial" than "cerebral," that it is oriented more toward the emotions than toward the intelligence. The counterpart of the *Organon,* Aristotle's *Rhetoric,* summit of the path that for a century Corax and Tisias, Gorgias and the Platonic *Phaedrus* had been blazing, is the technical treatise of the persuasive word.

The concern of Aristotle with the problem of verbal persuasion did not stop here. That concern, so Greek and so Platonic —the anti-Sophist Plato shared in it as fervently as did Sophism—is alive in some pages of the *Nicomachean Ethics* and of the *Politics* and in almost every page of the *Poetics*. As a word addressed to another human being, what else does the literary work seek than to persuade of something? And among all the literary genres is not the drama perhaps the one which most directly accomplishes that persuasive function? In my opinion the old, everlasting, and never solved problem of *katharsis*, to which the famous Aristotelian definition of tragedy refers, must be studied from this point of view.

In this chapter I shall attempt to set forth and interpret Aristotelian thought on the persuasive power of the word. The psychological aspects of the *Organon*—what Aristotle says and thinks about the psychological operation of the dialectical *logos*—in other words, the psychology of logical conviction, will occupy a subordinate place in my endeavor, and I shall study successively the doctrine of persuasion contained in the *Rhetoric* and the cathartic action of tragedy mentioned in the *Poetics*. It will not take us long to see that both inquiries are essentially connected with the abiding theme of this book, the therapy of the word.

I. I have just noted that the *Rhetoric* of Aristotle is the climax of a centuries-long enterprise marked by the names of Corax and Tisias, Gorgias and the *Phaedrus*.[3] But in that undoubtedly splendid culmination all the seeds contained in the work of those who had made it possible did not germinate. Aristotle says that his predecessors, mindful of the judicial or forensic type of oratory above all, gave up the cultivation of the other two, the deliberative (the oratory of political assemblies) and the apodictic or demonstrative. This is historically true, but it is also true that Gorgias, Antiphon, and Plato had

---

3. This enumeration is far from being complete; to it should be added the names of Lysias, Theodoros, Antiphon and Isocrates, the Platonic *Gorgias*, etc. An excellent synopsis of the history of rhetoric up to Aristotle can be read in the "Introduction" by A. Tovar to his edition of Aristotle's *Rhetoric* (*Aristóteles. Retórica*, Madrid, 1953).

begun the construction of a fourth type of persuasive word, the therapeutic or curative type, difficult to include in any of the three that Aristotle considers and never named by the philosopher. If the Aristotelian *Rhetoric* is viewed in this light, will we succeed in discovering in its body the gap to be filled by this unborn and possible fourth type of the *logos pithanos* or "persuasive speech"? Did there exist in Aristotle in masked form a speculative theory of verbal psychotherapy? Examining with care what the *Rhetoric* was, and methodically transferring its doctrine to the curative task of the psychotherapist, let us try to find out.

The *Rhetoric* of Aristotle is born of a purpose at once Platonic and anti-Platonic. Insofar as he is heir to a good part of the thought of the *Phaedrus*, *Philebus*, and *Laws*, and gives completion to the design openly or latently contained in those dialogues—the composition of an *Art of Rhetoric* that will be a true *technê* and even a true "science" or *epistêmê* (*Politics*, 304c–d)—Aristotle is a follower of Plato. But having set himself to accomplish his endeavor the pupil soon becomes aware that he cannot complete it without departing from his master on two essential points, one of moral character and the other of logical nature. In order to be a true *technê* rhetoric must place itself at a distance from morals: "its rule," writes M. Dufour, "is not of course immoralism, subversion against traditional morals, but amoralism, provisional indifference to the imperative."[4] The orator, in principle, should be technically able to persuade of a thing and of its opposite (*Rhet.*, I, 1, 1355, a 30). Nor is this all. In contrast to the Platonic warning against *doxa* or opinion—a warning only ignored by the Athenian philosopher when he thought that opinion could be set on the road to truth by means of "mythical speech"—Aristotle discovers that a science of the "likely" is also possible, and that this science is precisely rhetoric. The premises of rhetorical arguments have to be generally admitted opinions (*endoxa*) and common notions (*koina*). But rhetoric does not therefore nec-

---

4. Aristote. *Rhétorique*, I, 3 ("Introduction" to the edition of "Les Belles Lettres," Paris, 1932).

essarily go against the true and the good. The orator should be able to persuade of a thing and of its opposite, "but not in order to do both things, for one should not be persuaded to evil, but so that we may not be unaware of the way in which it is evil, and so that when another uses the same reasons we can undo them" (I, 1, 1355, a 31–34). The purpose of the orator and hence his intention decides the moral complexion of the rhetorical adroitness: "Sophism does not consist of ability but of intention" (I, 1, 1355, b 18). And on the other hand, "both to see the truth as well as to see the likely is characteristic of the same ability," and so the habit of conjecturing in regard to the likely is not essentially different from the habit of finding the true (I, 1, 1355, a 17–19). Finally, the dialectical *logos* and the rhetorical *logos* have the same subject, and between dialectic and rhetoric there is no opposition but rather correlation and a complementary relationship (I, 1, 1354, a 1). In contrast to Plato "Aristotle definitely accepts," A. Tovar correctly states, "that rhetoric does not endeavor merely to *dêloun* [to cause to see] but that it is legitimate for it also to *psychagôgein* [to lead souls], to which end one must study character and the passions. Perfecting dialectic and at the same time compromising with the traditional Sophistic positions in rhetoric he thereby achieves a true synthesis in which Sophism and Platonism are mingled." [5]

But with all this, what is rhetoric for Aristotle? It is—or, "let it be," as Aristotle says, in order to emphasize the relevance of the rhetorical theme to the area of opinion—"the capacity to consider in each case what there may be in it suitable for persuasion" (I, 2, 1355, b 25). The mission of rhetoric is hence not to persuade but to discover the persuasive element that

5. "Introduction," p. xxxi. The passages from the *Rhetoric* will be cited by me according to this version. The philological and philosophical problem of Aristotle's *Rhetoric* has won present-day currency since Fr. Solmsen (*Die Entwicklung der aristotelischen Logik und Rhetorik*, Berlin, 1929) applied to this work the genetic and stratigraphic method that W. Jaeger had applied to the *Metaphysics* and to other works of the Stagirite. This summary indication will suffice here. Anyone wishing to go deeply into the subject should see the above-mentioned "Introduction" by A. Tovar.

there may be in each case, just as the mission of medicine is not to cure—so put, in an absolute sense—but to ascertain how and in what measure each patient is curable (I, 1, 1355, b 10–15). In his own way Aristotle follows the idea of the parallelism between medicine and rhetoric that Plato set forth in the *Phaedrus*. But such a correlation does not exclude the more general character of rhetoric since the latter, unlike the other arts which have a particular and well-determined subject matter (medicine, health, and illness; geometry, the proportions of size; arithmetic, number), has as its object persuasion in respect to any given thing of which it may be possible to persuade (I, 2, 1355, b 23–35). One may ask accordingly: if the state of illness is in some measure modifiable by persuasion, can the existence of a therapeutic or curative genre in the body of rhetoric be denied?

As I have said, the classes that Aristotle distinguishes in the latter are three: the deliberative or political, the judicial or forensic, and the demonstrative or apodictic, and in the three the purpose of the discourse and the attitude of the hearer are different. In the deliberative type the purpose is the advantageous or the harmful, and the hearer, the member of the Assembly, is psychologically oriented toward the future; in the judicial type the end is the just or the unjust, and the hearer, the judge, primarily contemplates the past; in the demonstrative type the end is the beautiful or the ugly, and the hearer, the person who is being praised or blamed, takes into account the present above all.

In all types of rhetorical persuasion the orator uses arguments proper to his art to attain his goal. It is not by chance that these are called *pisteis:* as though we were to say "trusts" or "beliefs." Persuasion, *peithô,* and belief or faith, *pistis,* are in Greek, as we know, words derived from the same root. A man is persuaded when he believes what he is told. Hence that which persuades, the proof or argument of the persuasion, is also that in which one believes or has faith, *pistis*. And these "suasive arguments" or *pisteis* can be, says Aristotle, technical proofs, that is, belonging to the art of the orator, and nontechnical proofs, that is, proofs given to the orator in a manner prior and foreign to his art, such as witnesses and documents and objects of all kinds. For dialectical knowledge real things are before all "beings," *onta;* for rhetorical knowledge, things are primarily "suasive proofs," *pisteis.* Thus, Heidegger, bringing grist to his mill, could say that the *Rhetoric* of Aristotle is "the first systematic hermeneutic of the daily circumstance of being with others."

Let us now return to the possibility of a fourth *genus* of rhetorical persuasion, the therapeutic or curative type. If among the three Aristotelian or traditional types there is any close to it, it is without doubt the deliberative. The principal purpose of the deliberative orator is "the useful," *to sympheron* (I, 3, 1358, b 23; I, 6, 1362, a 18, etc.); now we already know that the word is repeatedly used in the *Corpus Hippocraticum* almost with the force of a technical term in order to designate the supreme criterion of therapeutic action.[6] Deliberative persuasion has as its object the possible, but not that which is possible by nature (*physei*), such as the fact that the oak grows from the acorn or that a bath is refreshing, nor that which is possible as a result of chance (*apo tychês*), such as meeting a friend whom one does not expect to see, but "the things that can depend upon us and whose reason for occurrence consists in us" (I, 4, 1359, a 38). And is not this also the object of medicine? Is it not stated in *On the Art* that the physician should abstain from touching patients for whose malady he is unable to do anything useful (L. 6, 26)? Virchow once wrote that "politics is medicine on a large scale." From the point of view of the relationship between therapeutic persuasion and deliberative or political persuasion it could also be said, in the Aristotelian manner, that medicine is politics on a small scale. Health, too, is found among the goods that for Aristotle make up "the useful" (I, 6, 1362, b 14).

According to the *Rhetoric* the art of the orator consists of

6. For the *sympheron* in the *Corpus Hippocraticum*—and more generally in the literature of the fifth century—see F. Heinimann, *Nomos und Physis,* pp. 128 ff.

making skillful use of the three cardinal technical proofs: the character of the speaker, the inclination of the hearer, and what is said in the speech (I, 2, 1356, a 1–5). Let us study then, from our point of view, these three principal factors of rhetorical persuasion and try to understand how Aristotle conceives of the effect of that which is heard upon the soul of the hearer.

The character (*êthos*) of the orator is "almost the principal one of the suasive proofs" (I, 2, 1356, a 13), especially in the case of deliberative oratory, because "we believe according to how the one that is speaking appears to be, that is, if he appears good or well intentioned or both" (I, 8, 1366, a 10–12). This "character" does not depend only on the natural qualities of the speaker, but on the moral habits that he may have acquired in the course of his life—probity (I, 2, 1356, a 13), prudence, virtue, kindness (II, 1, 1378, a 9)—and ultimately on the relationship established between him and his hearers: "for it is of great importance for persuasion, especially in deliberative oratory . . . how the orator presents himself and that the audience should suppose that he is in a certain frame of mind in regard to them, and moreover if they are in some way inclined in respect to him" (II, 1, 1377, a 25–29). The orator puts his character to test when he presents himself to his hearers and addresses them. The close moral relationship between them gives decisive timeliness and validity to what that character was; and so it occurs that on some occasions ignorant orators are more persuasive than the very learned and subtle, through being closer to their audience.

Now, all this is repeated with impressive parallelism in the relation between the physician and the patient. The character of the therapist—his natural qualities, his habits, his acquired virtues, his prestige—has considerable importance in the efficacy of his prescriptions, according to several Hippocratic writings: the *Prognosis, The Law, On the Physician, On Decorum*. That character is put into effect and operates when the physician comes into contact with his patient. Nor is it impossible in the practice of medicine, especially when the activity of the physician is psychotherapeutic, for the unlearned man to have more success than the scholar.

No less important to the efficacy of rhetorical persuasion is the disposition (*diathesis*) of the hearer. Plato had already taught (*Phaedrus*, 271a–272b) that the orator in his speeches must adhere to the various "aspects" (*eidê*) of the souls of those who listen to him. Now Aristotle applies the term *diathesis* to the occasional disposition of the soul in each one of its possible "aspects"—Galen will later say that disease is a "preternatural disposition" on the part of the one who suffers it, *diathesis para physin*—and sees such a "disposition" as determined by the passions (*pathê*) and the qualities (age, fortune, immoral and virtuous habits) of those hearing the speech. Especially the passions, for the character of men is actualized and revealed by them on every occasion. Persuasion, Aristotle says, is produced in the hearers "when they are drawn into a passion by the speech, for our judgments are not the same with grief as with happiness, with friendship as with hatred" (I, 2, 1356, a 15–16). This places Aristotle's mind before a double rhetorical problem: to define what a passion is and to explain how to modify or to provoke it.[7]

What is a passion? From the point of view of rhetoric the passions are "that because of which men change and differ in judgment, and which are followed by pain and pleasure; such as anger, pity, fear and the like, and their opposites" (II, 1, 1378, a 22–24). Acting upon the manner of judging, the passions play the most important part in the determination of the "opinions" of men. *The Nicomachean Ethics* will say that passion is a movement (*kinêsis*) and an alteration (*alloiôsis*) in the being of man (1105, b 19 ff); the treatise *de anima* will stress the essential participation of the body in the change of one who becomes impassioned (*de anima*, 403, a 16 ff). More than a simple affective state, *pathos* is for Aristotle a more or

---

7. "It is no accident," writes Heidegger, "that the first systematically developed interpretation of the emotions was not set forth in the frame of the *Psychology*. Aristotle investigates the *pathê* in the second book of the *Rhetoric*" (*Sein und Zeit*, 4th ed. Halle, 1935, p. 138).

less fleeting change in the being of one who experiences it, a change to which an alteration of the body and another in the way of judging and believing simultaneously belong.

But the orator cannot be satisfied with knowing what a passion is. As a *technitês* or technician of rhetoric, he needs to know also how to produce it and why he produces it. In order to arouse, quench, or modify a passion, in order to change the "disposition" of his audience, the orator must bear in mind the four data that constitute the subjective or moral proofs of persuasion: the particular disposition of the soul in each one of the passions (psychology of anger and calm, of love and hatred, of fear and valor, etc.), the persons in whose presence each passion is usually experienced, the occasions or situations in which each passion most frequently arises, and finally the various qualities of the audience according to their age, virtues, vices, and fortune (nobility, wealth, etc.) (II, 1, 1377, b 24–27, and II, 12, 1388, b 32–1389, a 2). In view of this fourfold reality—Aristotle carefully studies it step by step in chapters 2–17 of Book II—the orator must know how to produce in his hearers anger, calm, friendship, hatred, fear, and the other passions.

I wonder if this is not the case with the "physicianly orator" or healer by the word, such as Antiphon was in Corinth toward the end of the fifth century B.C., and such as are today those who call themselves psychotherapists. Let us restrict ourselves to the letter of Aristotle's *Rhetoric*. According to it, is not disease a cause of anger? (II, 2, 1379, a 15.) And on the other hand cannot anger be a cause of disease? Without a broad and precise knowledge of those four subjective proofs of persuasion, without a clear and detailed idea about the seven motives of human actions—fortune, nature, violence, custom, reflexion, choleric appetite, and lustful appetite (I, 10, 1369, a 6–8)—and without distinguishing with care among the various appetites the irrational or spontaneous, and the rational or elicited (I, 11, 1370, a 19–27), there is no possibility of being an orator "according to art," nor of technically practicing verbal psychotherapy. Even from a merely psychotherapeutic point of view no one will judge this shrewd observation of Aristotle on fear to be pointless: "neither are they afraid who already believe that the worst has happened to them and they are indifferent to the future . . . for in order to be afraid, it is necessary that there remain some hope of salvation in respect to that which is tormenting [*agôniôsin*] us" (II, 5, 1383, a 3–6).

All this—the character of the speaker, the disposition of the listener—is extremely important to the orator, but the decisive matter will always be what he says in his speech, the third of the three technical proofs that Aristotle distinguishes, for "the listeners believe in the speech when we show the truth or what appears to be the truth with it, according to what is persuasive in each particular case" (I, 2, 1356, a 20–21). In rhetoric too the *logos* is always above the *êthos*. It cannot be surprising that it is in the explanation of this persuasive proof that the personal contribution of Aristotle to rhetoric turns out to be most abundant and important: Aristotle was, as we know, the inventor of the discipline that we today call "logic." A whole series of types of arguments—the enthymeme, a syllogism of probability or rhetorical syllogism; the example, a rhetorical form of induction; the maxim or assertion in respect to that with which actions have to do and which can be chosen or avoided in acting; the citing of commonplace topics or bromides—and, in addition, a careful study of rhetorical elocution and of the external and internal form of the speech (Book III), comprise the Aristotelian doctrine of persuasive speech. I do not believe it pertinent to set forth here in more detail the structure of this central body of the *Rhetoric;* nor is that more detailed explanation necessary to discover that the enthymemes, examples, maxims, topics, good locution, and good composition, all filled, of course, with the contents that the concrete individual nature of the case being dealt with demands, constitute the most important part of the catalogue of devices that verbal psychotherapy utilizes. The psychotherapist, like Monsieur Jourdain with prose, turns out Aristotelian rhetoric without knowing it. A "rhetorical" analysis of any of the clinical histories of Freud would clearly show this.

We finally come to the fourth and last of the theories proposed above: the way that Aristotle understands the action of the persuasive word in the soul of the one on whom it works. Here is a man persuaded by a skillful speech. What has happened in his soul? Aristotle tries to understand the mechanism of psychological transformation by means of five principal concepts: character (*êthos*), disposition (*diathesis*), passion (*pathos*), opinion (*doxa*), and belief (*pistis, peithô*). In the rhetorical encounter—that of the orator with his hearer—two characters, that of the speaker and that of the listener, are placed in mutual connection. As a consequence of that personal contact, simultaneously intellectual and affective, the soul and character of the hearer take on a particular disposition pertaining to one or another of the passions. Acting upon them with the devices of his art the orator modifies them according to the ends toward which his speech is composed; by means of the influence exerted by the passion on the way of seeing and judging things he promotes in his hearer a set of new opinions or a change in his former opinions. In other words the listener is persuaded of something; this is the same as saying, since to be persuaded is ultimately to believe, that in the soul of the hearer new beliefs have appeared, old beliefs have undergone a process of modification, or dormant beliefs have come into force. In all this a decisive role is taken by the enlightenment with respect to itself that the soul of the hearer acquires. Indeed, the word of the orator leads the hearer to see reality and himself in a hitherto unrealized way and at times reveals to him zones of his own life the existence of which he did not suspect before.

And all this to what purpose? The technique of the orator can in principle serve both an end and its opposite. But if his intention is honest and he adheres to that which the nature of the art and the nature of man demand, his ends cannot be other than truth, goodness, and happiness. The nature of the art demands these ends, for "the true and the good are naturally of better knit reasoning and more persuasive" (I, 1, 1355, a 37–39), and the nature of man also demands them because happiness (*eudaimonia*) "is the object in view of which each man in particular and all in common choose or reject"; the reason for which "persuasions and dissuasions are always about happiness and the things that tend toward it or about their opposites" (I, 5, 1360, b 4–11). The *sôphrosynê* that the *logos kalos* of Socrates in the Platonic *Charmides* had as its goal does not seem to be very far away from the *eudaimonia* that speech according to art should produce, in the *Rhetoric* of Aristotle.

I repeat once more my question: could not what Aristotle says of deliberative, demonstrative, and judicial persuasion be easily transferred to therapeutic persuasion? In the psychotherapeutic meeting, too, a more or less harmonious collision occurs between the character of the physician and that of the patient; in that of the latter and in his disposition, which now receives the name of illness, there are for definite reasons some passions or others predominant as well; the psychotherapist also endeavors to modify them in accordance with the ends proposed in each session; too, the medical treatment continually elicits in the patient new opinions and beliefs, while at the same time it enlightens and illuminates him in respect to himself; too, finally, happiness—now in the form of health, one of the parts of *eudaimonia* (I, 5, 1361, b 3–7)—is the end to which the therapy is designed. The addition of a fourth *genus* to the body of the *Rhetoric* of Aristotle does not seem to be a gratuitous and unfounded notion.

II. In the work of Aristotle the power of the word is primarily persuasion, but not persuasion alone. In a famous passage of the *Poetics* that power receives the name of *katharsis*. As the mention of poetic catharsis comes to the fore in another and no less famous passage of the *Politics*, I shall begin by transcribing it. Aristotle is discussing the usefulness of music in the education of the young and remarks as follows:

> We admit the division of melodies established by some philosophers, classifying them as ethical, practical and enthusiastic and attributing to each of these classes a particular kind of harmony, and we assert on the other hand that

music should be studied not because it bestows a single benefit but many, since it should be cultivated with education and purification [*katharsis*] in view—when we deal with poetics we shall explain with more clarity what we mean by the term purification, which we are now simply using—; in the third place, it should be cultivated also as an amusement and as recreation and relaxation after labor. It is evident accordingly that all harmonies should be used but not all in the same way; the ethical predominantly for education, the practical and enthusiastic, performed by others, for audition as well. For the passions that take on great vehemence in some souls, such as pity, fear and enthusiasm, exist in all with differences of degree. Some people even have a tendency to allow themselves to be overcome by the last named, and so we see that when they make use of the melodies that enrapture the soul, sacred music affects them as though they found in it healing and purification [*katharsis*]. Those who are possessed by compassion and terror or, in general, by any passion, and other persons to the degree that each is affected by these emotions, necessarily must have this same experience, and thus in all there will be produced a certain purification [*katharsis*] and relief accompanied by pleasure. In an analogous way cathartic melodies also inspire an innocent happiness in men (*Polit.*, VIII, 7, 1341, b 32–1342, a 16).[8]

The passage of the *Poetics* to which I refer is the definition of tragedy; the latter is, according to Aristotle,

the imitation of a lofty and complete action, of adequate length, in language embellished within its own medium in conformity to its various parts, performed by persons in action and not by means of narration, and which by means of pity and fear accomplishes the purging [*katharsis*] of such passions. I call "embellished language" that which has

8. I am quoting from the translation by Julián Marías and María Araujo, *Aristóteles. Política* (Madrid, 1951).

rhythm, melody and is uttered in song, and I say "in conformity to its various parts" because certain of them are performed with the aid of metre while others are uttered in song (*Poet.*, 6, 1449, b 24-31).

Like all poetry, tragedy is imitation, *mimêsis;* but it is distinguished from the other poetic genres by the nature of the object imitated (a lofty or valiant human action), by the medium made use of for the imitation (combining them all: discourse, harmony, and rhythm), by the manner of carrying out the mimetic design (action of the characters of the drama, instead of narration), but above all by the fact that it produces in the spectator a specific pleasure (*hêdonê*) and a purgation or purification (*katharsis*) of the two passions that the tragic spectacle arouses in the soul: pity and fear.

The words in which the action of the tragic poem is expressed have, then, a particular power that Aristotle calls purgation, purification, or catharsis. What was this tragic catharsis in the thought of Aristotle? Is the supposed cathartic action of tragedy related in any way to medicine and, more concretely, to the therapy of the word? Such are our problems at this point.

Delicate, enigmatic, and interminable is this question of tragic catharsis. "There can hardly be in universal literature a passage of equal length on which such a deluge of works has poured down," says Gudeman in his critical edition of the *Poetics*.[9] "In Greek literature there is no more famous passage than the ten words of the *Poetics* relative to catharsis," writes Hardy in the prologue to his edition.[10] From the writers of the Italian Renaissance (Robortello, Vettori, Minturno, Castelvetro), the French and German preceptors of the seventeenth and eighteenth centuries (Batteux, Chapelain, Scudéry, Lessing) down to to our day, passing through the decisive works of J. Bernays and H. Weil at the height of the nineteenth century, there was not a moment of rest for the pens of philolo-

---

9. A. Gudeman, *Aristoteles. Poetik* (Berlin and Leipzig, 1934), p. 167.
10. J. Hardy, *Aristote. Poétique* (Paris, 1932), p. 16.

gists. Hardly had the study by Bernays been published than it gave rise to no less than one hundred and fifty works for or against it; and already in 1856, a year before it appeared, the good Don Juan Valera wrote of the Aristotelian definition of tragedy: "words of Aristotle that everyone understands in his own way." [11]

It would not be difficult to compose a history of European feeling and thought following the thread of this immense philological and exegetical hodgepodge. The Renaissance commentators were accustomed to interpret the favorable effect of tragic catharsis as a hardening to the vicissitudes of life produced by familiarity with spectacles that fill us with fear and compassion. The French preceptors and playwrights of the seventeenth century, more devout, extend the cathartic process to all the passions and interpret it as a purification of the individual. Corneille, for example, thinks that the spectacle of tragedy moves us "to purge, moderate, rectify and even eradicate in ourselves the passion that, before our eyes, plunges the persons whom we pity into misfortune." [12] In the seventeenth century a new hermeneutic attitude first appears. The medical definition of the word *katharsis* begins to be recalled and is understood from the point of view of individual happiness and well-being. Batteux holds that "tragedy gives us the terror and compassion that please us, and eliminates from them that excessive degree or that mixture of horror that displeases us." Attention is centered now on the "happiness without mixture of pain" that Aristotle deems the proper purpose of cathartic melodies. And presently, well in the nineteenth century and under the influence of positivism, there begins in the interpretation of the Aristotelian text the period which we may well call "modern." As I have said, Jacob Bernays was its principal initiator.[13]

Supported by a minute analysis of the text from the *Politics*

11. J. Valera, *Obras Completas* (Editorial Aguilar, Madrid, 1942), 2, 73.
12. P. Corneille, *Les grands écrivains de la France* (Paris, 1862), *1*, 53.
13. The study of Bernays appeared for the first time in the Mémoires of the Academy of Breslau in 1857 and was subsequently reprinted in

transcribed above, by the passage of Iamblichus' work, *De mysteriis*, in which he views tragic catharsis as a discharge of emotions both repressed and heightened by repression, by the commentary of Proclus on Plato's *Republic,* and, of course, by the writings of the *Corpus Hippocraticum,* Bernays boldly breaks with the moral interpretation of Aristotle's definition and understands "catharsis of the passions" as a purging of the soul in the most purely medical sense of this term. "Concretely taken," he writes, "the word *katharsis* means one of the following two things in Greek: *either* the expiation of a guilt by means of certain priestly rites, *or* the suppression or relief of a disease by a purgative medical remedy." Aristotle would have adhered exclusively to this second definition; hence his aesthetic theory had no moral character, as was generally believed before Bernays, nor a hedonistic character, as Ed. Müller had thought; the term "catharsis" in the Aristotelian definition would be merely "a designation transferred from the somatic to the affective in order to designate to the treatment of a sufferer a treatment with which the endeavor is not made to transform or repress the aggrieving element but to excite and foster it in order thus to bring about the relief of the sufferer." The purgative agent would produce an aggravation of the disturbance in the humor causing the malady, and this increase in intensity of the disturbance would provoke the expulsion or "discharge" of the excessive matter and reestablish the physical equilibirum. Similar, in their way, would be the action of "enthusiastic" melodies. The catharses of the passions could be ultimately reduced to a "homeopathic" treatment of the spectator of the tragedy, at the end of which the latter, "cured" according to the principle of *similia similibus,* would gain relief accompanied by pleasure.[14]

Despite the abundant discussion of which it has been the

Zwei Abhandlungen über die Aristotelische Theorie des Drama (Berlin, 1880). Parallel to this interpretation by Bernays and independent of it is that of H. Weil, which was presented by its author under the title of *Ueber die Wirkung der Tragödie nach Aristoteles* at the 10th Assembly of German Philologists (Basel, 1848).

14. Pp. 12, 16, 64, 65, and 92. Italics (*entweder . . . oder*) are Bernays'.

object, Bernays' interpretation, M. Pohlenz wrote not long ago, has succeeded in creating a "common ground" for all the ensuing philological investigation.[15] But on this ground the debate on Aristotelian *katharsis* has continued without rest. I am not going to follow it in all detail, yet to point out the main viewpoints that have arisen here may perhaps not be without use. I seem to see three: in a certain number of those with opinions the accent of the interpretation is rather an *aesthetic* character; others adopt a hermeneutic position in which a *moral* point of view is clearly dominant; in the judgment of a third group, finally, the *medical* consideration of the problem is preponderant. I may be permitted, in accordance with the theme of my study, to limit my commentary to this final position.[16]

Shortly after the first version of Bernays' work had been

15. M. Pohlenz, "Furcht und Mitleid? Ein Nachwort," *Hermes, 84* (1956), 60.

16. Among the representatives of the most *aesthetic* orientation can be mentioned E. Howald ("Eine vorplatonische Kunsttheorie," *Hermes, 54* (1919), 187–207); A. Rostagni (*Aristotele. Poetica*, 2d ed. Torino, 1945); M. K. Lienhard (*Zur Entstehung und Geschichte von Aristoteles Poetik*, Diss. Zurich, 1950); and H. Koller (*Die Mimesis in der Antike*, Bern, 1954). According to them Aristotle, supported by the old musical doctrine of the Pythagoreans, would have freed poetry from the rhetorical exclusiveness with which Gorgias had conceived it.

There are not a few authors in whom the moral point of view, more or less religiously, psychologically, or metaphysically conceived, is prevalent. Catharsis, rather than a "purging" or "sifting"—*diakrisis*, as Plato would say—is now a "purification" or "cleansing," in short an "improving," of one who undergoes it. I shall cite among them F. Susemihl (*Aristoteles. Ueber die Dichtkunst*, Leipzig, 1874, and *Aristoteles. Politik*, Leipzig, 1879); M. Untersteiner (*Origine della Tragedia*, Milan 1942); A. Tumarkin, ("Die Kunsttheorie von Aristoteles im Rahmen seiner Philosophie," *Mus. Hel., 2* [1945], 108); E. P. Papanoutsos ("La catharsis Aristotélicienne," *Eranos, 46* [1948], 77, and "La catharsis des passions d'après Aristote," *Collections de l'Institut Français d'Athènes*, 1953, p. 26); K. H. Volkmann-Schluck ("Die Lehre von der Katharsis in der *Poetik* des Aristoteles," *Varia Variorum*, Festgabe für K. Reinhardt, 1952, p. 104); H. Weinstock (*Die Tragödie des Humanismus*, Heidelberg, 1953); R. Schottländer ("Eine Fessel der Tragödiedeutung," *Hermes, 81* [1953], 22); R. Stark ("Aristotelesstudien," *Zetemata, 8* [1954], 37); and K. v. Fritz ("Tragische Schuld und poetische Gerechtigheit in der griechische Tragödie," *Studium Generale, 8* [1955], 235). An important feature of the mentality brought about by World War I published, A. Döring [17] undertook a detailed study of the *Corpus Hippocraticum* in order to confirm with documentary proof the knotty problem of Bernays' argument. According to the latter, traditional medical doctrine in Greece taught that a purgative acts by first exacerbating and even bringing to a paroxysm the disease that it subsequently is to cure; that is what, psychologically, the effect of the religious songs of "enthusiastic" nature to which the passage in the *Politics* refers must have been, and the effect of tragedy as well with respect to the passions aroused by the tragic spectacle in the soul of the spectator. But Döring could only carry out his endeavor by forcing the meaning of the verbs *kinein* (to move) and *agein* (to act) with which the *Hippocratic Collection* customarily designates the action of purges, and by gratuitously supposing that those two terms, especially the first, usually have in the *Corpus* the same sense as *tarachê* (disturbance) and *tarattein* (to disturb or to trouble).

The recent excellent study by Jeanne Croissant was more subtle and discriminating.[18] Mlle. Croissant's interpretation, which coincides with that of Bernays on fundamental issues, differs from it on two important points, the first having to do with the origin and the significance of the word *katharsis* and the second relating to the purgative action of cathartic agents. In the opinion of this author Aristotle must have added a new sense to those previously possessed by that word: "Aristotle, by using the term *katharsis* to designate the role that he attributed to pathetic music, enriched with a new metaphorical sense a concept of already very widely varying aspects" (63). But this does not exclude the philosopher from having taken the word from religious language, within which it was used to

---

and not subsequently eliminated (antipositivism, irrationalism, return to metaphysics, neo-romanticism) is expressed in this moral and religious view of Attic tragedy and of the catharsis of the passions that Aristotle attributed to the tragedy.

17. *Die Kunstlehre des Aristoteles* (Jena, 1876). Likewise Bernaysian is the attitude of Bywater in his *Aristotle on the Art of Poetry* (Oxford, 1909).

18. *Aristote et les mystères* (Liège et Paris, 1932).

designate very diverse ritual "purifications." A passage from the *Politics* gives clear indication of this: "The flute is not an instrument of moral character but rather of orgiastic nature, so that it should be used on those occasions in which the spectacle aims more at purification [*katharsis*] than instruction" (1341, a 21-22). The allusion of Aristotle to the orgiastic rites, Dionysiac or Corybantic, cannot be clearer. Now that passage is merely a page prior to the one that Bernays so ably and pertinently cited. Moreover, Bernays plainly errs in the interpretation of the passage where Proclus discusses the theory of Aristotle on the effect of tragedy and with this error of his ultimately confirms the derivation of that word.[19] But if the term *katharsis* in the *Politics* and the *Poetics* has a religious origin, its meaning no longer possesses such a character: *katharsis* now means the "purgation" of the passions that the hearing of enthusiastic music and the viewing of tragedy commonly arouse. The religious "enthusiasm" and the tragic spectacle must have had the same working mechanism, of cathartic or purgative nature. This brings us to the second point of the disagreement between J. Croissant and Bernays: that relating to the mechanism of musical and tragic purgation.

That mechanism must be of psychophysiological character, and even purely physiological and somatic; the psychology of

19. In his *Commentary on the Republic* (I, p. 42, 1.12, p. 50 passim) Proclus defines the effect that Aristotle attributed to tragedy not as a *katharsis* but as an *aphosiôsis* of the passions and then contradicts the author of the *Poetics* by stating that the ideas maintained by him do not correspond to the usual sense of the term *aphosiôsis* (purification or expiation). Therefore Aristotle must also have used this word. Bernays admits that the Stagirite really used the term, but he imagines that he used it with the metaphorical and profane sense of mere "adjustment" or "accommodation": adjustment or accommodation of the passions (*Abfinde der Affekte*). In this he is in error, according to J. Croissant: in the classical period *aphosiôsis* only had two senses: one direct, religious, and the other metaphysical, "to do something to pacify the conscience" (Isaeus, Plato), in no way an "accommodation of the passions." All this indicates that, contrary to Bernays' opinion, Aristotle drew those two words—*katharsis*, *aphosiôsis*—from a religious source. Rohde (*Psyche*, 13, 3) is of the same opinion in respect to the Platonic use of the word *katharsis*.

Aristotle is always psychophysiological (44), and the Aristotelian explanation of religious phenomena, in this case enthusiasm, does not depart from this rule. A very fine and detailed examination of *Problem* XXX, 1—whose teaching is for Mlle. Croissant totally Aristotelian—should give the key to the enigma. Indeed, according to this *Problem* a whole broad series of very diverse phenomena—the successive psychological effects of wine, the results of the sex act and purges upon melancholic subjects, musical and religious enthusiasm—have for Aristotle a common somatic substratum, of which process the economy of animal heat and the physiology of black bile are principal parts. This must be the reason why melancholy individuals whose black bile is neither very warm nor very cold are outstanding in education, philosophy, politics and the arts (*Problem*, 954, a 38–b 4). J. Croissant writes:

> Aristotle found the elements that were to give birth to his theory: the close relation between inebriation and enthusiasm and, on the other hand, an attempted explanation describing in accordance with mechanical laws a process analogous to that which he had observed in melancholy drunkards.[20] These two phenomena were by nature destined to unite in the spirit of Aristotle. Their association was the more imperative inasmuch as the facts of religious psychology that the philosopher sought to explain commonly bore the names of *katharsis* and *katharmos*. This gave rise to another approximation, no less necessary in one who was searching for a physiological explanation; because medi-

20. Plato writes in the *Laws* in regard to what occurs in Bacchic enthusiasm: "When someone applies mild external agitation to states of this sort, the motion coming from without is juxtaposed to that within, which is terrible and violent, and dominates it; and when it has done so produces peace and calm in the soul, freeing her from the tormenting palpitation of the heart, a thing much to be desired. The motion sends the children to sleep and as for the others, who remain awake and dance to the pipe with the help of the gods to whom they offer acceptable sacrifices, we see that soundness of mind is substituted for their frenzy; this explanation, even though we have expressed it in so few words, has some persuasive power" (790e, 791b).

cal *katharsis*, the direct treatment of melancholy individuals, led to the same soothing result . . . The comparison by Aristotle:—as though they found in it [in sacred music] healing and purgation (*Politics*, 1342, a 10–11)—thus has a general scope that goes beyond the mere idea of a medical purgation to which the first view of the text seems to lead. If the Stagirite has expressed himself in such a manner it is because he was attempting to retain the original and religious term of *katharsis*, transferring it purely and simply to the physiological realm. Nothing reveals better the origin of the term of which he has made use . . . The word *katharsis* had the double advantage of recalling the picture in which the healing of enthusiasm and its religious interpretation occurred, and of being in the work of Aristotle a synthetic formula designating a physiological phenomenon. In his opinion the effect of wine, the purge, and the sex act were three different manners of purgation, the results of which would be identical in the melancholy . . . With this set of data Aristotle constructed his doctrine of psychic catharsis: catharsis of enthusiasm by the spectacle of the mysteries, and of other passions by that of the secular theatre . . . In his criticism of the theatre Plato had adopted the position of the moralizing statesman. But if Aristotle demanded less of man he was not for all that less a moralist, for he was a philosopher and never lost view of the ideal of good living [*to eu zên*] . . . When they are not harmful—thinks Aristotle—pleasures serve the ultimate end as much as does repose, and the pleasure of the theater is one of them. (104, 105, 110).

Such, in outline, is the interpretation by Mlle. Croissant. Let us freely grant its merits, but let us not overlook its limitation. The psychology of Aristotle is *always* physiological. True. But being *always* physiological, in the sense that this latter word has today, is it *only* physiological? Such, as we shall see, is the key to the insufficiency of this excellently elaborated interpretation of the Aristotelian idea of *katharsis*.[21]

The hermeneutical attitude of M. Kommerell in his book *Lessing und Aristoteles* is also Bernaysian.[22] After studying the history of interpretations of the Aristotelian text up to Lessing and Goethe the author sets forth his personal point of view. A detailed formal and material analysis of the genitive that depends upon the word *katharsis* in the Aristotelian definition—"catharis *of* compassion and fear"—would show its quality as a "genitive of separation." Kommerell thinks that "compassion" had in Aristotle's mind more importance than "fear," and that one and the other constitute together a "disturbance" of the soul of the spectator. Thus "the psychological action of tragedy" is conceived of as a "complete purgation of the soul of disturbing emotions"—the separative character of the genitive indicated above has this sense—and the process of catharsis, analogous to that of a therapeutical remedy, remains "outside any category of values" (265 ff).

A careful philological study led F. Dirlmeier [23] to the same grammatical thesis: the genitive that expresses the operation of *katharsis* is separative; hence tragic catharsis would eliminate from the soul not only the compassion and fear that are disturbing it, but the other passions as well.[24] But Dirlmeier

21. P. Boyancé (*Le culte des Muses*, pp. 186 ff) has called attention to the fact that the "physiological" explanation of enthusiasm discovered by Jeanne Croissant does not indicate that it had no religious and divine character in the eyes of Aristotle. Black bile—"this is its essential character," says Mlle. Croissant, glossing Aristotle—has in itself a "pneumatic power"; now "the *pneuma* is the ether that Aristotle had defined in *Peri philosophias* as a fifth element (*pempton sôma*) of divine nature, which would constitute the substance of the stars and would bestow upon them its divinity. Aristotle has retained this theory." But aside from these reasons of religious character, others of psychological order demonstrate the limitation of Mlle. Croissant's thesis. We shall soon become acquainted with them.

22. M. Kommerell, *Lessing und Aristoteles* (Frankfurt am Main, 1940). A. Lesky has published a valuable critical review of this work in *Gnomon*, 17 (1941), 241 ff.

23. F. Dirlmeier, "Katharsis pathêmatôn," *Hermes*, 75 (1940), 81 ff.

24. According to this the famous passage should be translated: tragedy

goes farther and in the course of his work maintains these two bold theses: 1. The catharses of the *Politics* and of the *Poetics* are not similar but identical to one another; both must be purely musical; tragedy produces a cathartic effect inasmuch as music is part of it. 2. The literal text of Book VIII of the *Politics*—within which these two series of words: "game-education-amusement" and "catharsis-education-amusement" appear to be equivalent—would oblige one to think that the *katharsis* of which Aristotle speaks is completely outside the realm of *paideia* (education) and *diagôgê* (amusement of the adult after work), hence outside the area of the ethical (*êthicon*), and with *paidia* (game or pastime) belongs to the sphere of pleasure (*hêdonê*). But Pohlenz rightly asks: can one who like Aristotle has called the action that tragedy imitates "valiant" or "lofty" (*spoudaia*) call its most characteristic process a "game" or "pastime"? Aeschylus would have felt it to be blasphemy for anyone to consider his deeply religious interpretation of the victory of Salamis as *paidia*. And Sophocles and Euripides would have no better tolerated their personal labor in respect to the problem of parricide being characterized as a *game*. Not a single word in all the *Poetics* authorizes us to suppose that Aristotle considered tragedy as simple *paidia*.[25]

I must now comment upon a recent and important work by Wolfgang Schadewaldt.[26] In the interpretation of the inexhaustible Aristotelian text—"by means of compassion and fear tragedy accomplishes the catharsis of such passions"—what the genitive "of the passions," the pronoun "such," and the noun "catharsis" mean in it has been discussed. Now: why not begin the analysis by trying to understand what that "fear" (*phobos*) and that "compassion" (*eleos*) were in the mind of Aristotle? And above all: can the *phobos* and the *eleos* of the

---

effects the purgation "of *such* passions" ("such" in the sense of these and the others) and not "of said passions." Pohlenz holds the same opinion: the Greek text does not say *toutôn* but *toioutôn*.

25. M. Pohlenz, p. 69.
26. W. Schadewaldt, "Furcht und Mitleid?" *Hermes*, 83 (1955), 129 ff.

The Power of the Word in Aristotle

Aristotelian definition legitimately be translated by "fear" and "compassion"? The tragic catharsis purges the soul of the spectator; but from what does the latter really purge or free himself? Such was the point of departure of Schadewaldt.

His reply is for the moment negative. "Fear" is an extremely weak word by which to translate *phobos;* "compassion" is a term too much influenced by the moral sensibility of Christianity to express faithfully the real sense of *eleos. Phobos* should be translated as *Schrecken* (fright or horror) or as *Schauder* (shuddering or dread); *eleos* properly means *Jammer* (wretchedness) or *Rührung* (emotion, stirring up of the emotions). Both are elemental psychosomatic affections, not "higher" passions. The simple modern spectator to whom a play "gives goose flesh" and whom "it makes shed tears" until he soaks his handkerchief through would be closer to the reality that Aristotle sought to describe so accurately.

In consequence, the Aristotelian *katharsis* should be understood without recourse to motives or demands of, as it is usually put, a "higher" order, and by seeing in it only an elemental psychosomatic process. The proper effect of tragic catharsis is not moral: it is purely and simply pleasure (*hêdonê*), the pleasure for which attending the spectacle of tragedy specifically is designed. The *ergon* of the drama, what the tragic spectacle does and produces in one who views it, is a pleasure, and in the latter the psychosomatic "purgation" of which the *katharsis* consists has its ultimate effect. In this sense the doctrine of Bernays could not be more correct. When Aristotle was writing his famous definition he was not thinking of referring particularly or remotely to a purifying, improving, educative, or moral effect of *katharsis;* faithful to his purpose of "determining or delimiting the essence" (*horos tês ousias*) of the Attic tragedy he was attempting only to characterize accurately and truly the pleasure and the happiness that tragedy specifically produces.[27]

27. Schadewaldt, who disagrees with Bernays on not a few points of importance (p. 167, note 1), gives a synoptic table of recent attitudes toward *katharsis,* which I believe it useful to transcribe. It is as follows:

Now for Aristotle as for Plato (*Philebus*, 32a–b; *Tim.*, 64d) pleasure is primarily the return of the organism from a state of disturbance to the harmony proper to its particular nature, harmony *kata physin*. And is not this precisely what occurs in the human organism as a result of purgation by medicaments and after the excitement of Dionysiac and Corybantic enthusiasm? The well-being that the action of a purgative medicine produces, the calm following religious enthusiasm, and the pleasure caused by viewing a tragedy are not only "purgative pleasures" (*Purgierungs-Lüste*) but also—and this is extremely important—"harmless pleasures," "innocent pleasures" (*unschädliche Lüste*). Thus Aristotle understood it, and thus he puts it to everyone who can read, placing in mutual relation Chapter VI of the *Poetics* and Book VII of the *Politics*. With this the philosopher accomplishes two main purposes: to do away with political distrust of the drama on the part of Plato and to delimit precisely and strictly the "essence" of tragedy. For the Greeks poetry and art moved within the

---

A. The genitive that the word *katharsis* takes is an *objective* genitive. In this case there are two possibilities:
1. The effects of the fear and pity are "purified" in themselves. In such a case, "to purify" means to draw the emotions to "the just mean" (Lessing) or "to the purity of their essence" (Volkmann—Schluck); or to bring these passions from an irrational, undisciplined and confused state to another state that is rational, moderate, mutually harmonious and in harmony with the whole soul (Papanoutsos); or, finally, "purification" refers to the crude *hêdonê* elicited by *eleos* and *phobos*, makes it "innocent" and lifts it from the lowly realms of sensibility to the heights of spiritual good (Rostagni).
2. The purification does not pertain to the emotions themselves but to the harmful consequences, impressions and alterations—*pathêmata*—that they leave in the soul; the latter would thus, as it were, be "detoxified" (R. Stark).
B. The genitive ruled by the word *katharsis* is a *genitive of separation*. And in this case, two attitudes:
1. The soul through catharsis becomes free and cured of the "disturbances" that fear and, above all, pity—excessive sensitivity, irritability —bring with them (Krommerell).
2. Neither of the two emotions is eliminated, they merely remain free of their harmful excess, and man thus is improved (Pohlenz).
C. The arousing of fear and pity is only a means to free the soul from other passions or from an excess of them (Schottländer).

realm of the beautiful; the beautiful in its turn belonged to the sphere of the pleasurable; and in the case of tragedy the pleasurable had its place in the elemental and profound love of man for the terrible and moving. Homer had already spoken in the *Iliad* (XXIV, 507) of the "desire to weep," and the most spontaneous popular usage has coined in all languages a significant pleasurable sense of the adverbs "terribly" and "tremendously": nowadays any beautiful or desirable reality can be "terribly" nice or attractive. Conceived of in Aristotle's way, the characteristic pleasure of the tragic spectacle would ultimately be, in short, "a vital power, sensible and spiritual at the same time, embracing the whole reality of man" (160).

Tragic catharsis, contrary to what Dirlmeier asserts, is not merely an effect of music but is the effect of the whole action of the drama, as Aristotle himself was careful to note (*Poet.*, 1453, b 5). Throughout the course of the drama the psychic excitation of the spectator keeps rising along a "unitary curve," until, the dread and grief of his soul having reached the highest tension, the "purging" of those two passions is produced and the pleasurable relief of which the *hêdonê* of tragedy consists is attained. The spectator returns home "better," not in respect to his moral life but rather in relation to his physical well-being. This is very important to Aristotle, not as a *technikos* or writer of treatises on poetics but as a theoretician of urban life, for as Goethe once said, if the literary work does not have "moral purposes," save that of its own perfection, it does not for that reason cease to have "moral consequences." The labors and the tensions of daily work—the harsh *ascholia*, the *nec-otium* of the Latins—bring man distress (*lypai*), and there is nothing like the pleasure of tragedy to assuage it. Aristotle neatly marks out the boundaries of catharsis from education and instruction (*Polit.*, 1341, a 22); tragedy hence does not pursue ethical ends of itself, yet by the promotion of its characteristic pleasure it can and does accomplish, despite Plato, valuable political purposes.

Schadewaldt's line of argument, so powerful and skillful, has found a valuable follower in the young H. Flashar and a severe critic in the old Max Pohlenz. Flashar [28] set about studying, in Gorgias, Plato, the *Corpus Hippocraticum,* and Aristotle, what the "dread" (*phobos*) and the "grief" (*eleos*) that tragic catharsis effects were in their concrete psychosomatic reality. Shuddering, trembling, palpitations of the heart, and gooseflesh belong to the usual description of the first; the second is expressed by wailing and tears. *Phobos* and its symptoms, according to the *Corpus Hippocraticum,* are the consequence of an excessive "coldness" of the body, while tears, the principal sign of *eleos,* come from an excessive organic "moisture." Aristotle says essentially the same thing. The writings of the Stagirite on natural science teach that dread, *phobos,* is conceived as a "coldness of the excretions, residual or secretory" (*katapsyxis perittômatikê*). This permits one to infer for grief, *eleos,* the concept of an "excrementitious moistness" (*hygrotês perittômatikê*), an expression that appears in Aristotle, although not with immediate reference to *eleos.* All this would confirm the ideas of Schadewaldt: *phobos* and *eleos* are "dread" and "grief." The abnormal "coldness" that gives rise according to the physicians to *phobos* becomes concrete and real in the shivering that seizes the spectator of tragedy; and the *eleos,* a result of excessive organic "moisture," is for its part the emotion that puts tears in his eyes. To say then that the *katharsis* of tragedy is analogous to the *katharsis* of medicine would not be saying enough. What Aristotle asserts is that the tragic spectacle produces in the body a "purgation" in the most strictly medical sense of this word: the organism in fact is *materially* purged of the excess of cold and moistness disturbing it, a normal balance of these two qualities is thereupon reestablished within it, and a pleasant feeling of relief is born. The genitive of the Aristotelian definition cannot be other than "separative." Flashar however does not believe that his investigation has solved all the problems that that definition raises; therefore, he cautiously concludes, those "that do not pertain directly to the group of questions dealt with" should continue to be investigated.

28. His work has already been mentioned in Chapter 3.

I have purposely left for this place, last but not least, reference to the ideas of Max Pohlenz. Concern for the matter now under discussion is certainly of long standing with him,[29] but in his already mentioned reply to Schadewaldt's study this old master of classical philology has been the last to make public his opinion of tragic *katharsis*. More than once his ideas—also, of course, of Bernaysian origin—will appear in the pages to follow. I wish for the moment to limit myself to stating the quintessence of some of his objections to the philologist of Tübingen. Here, listed numerically, are those that appear most important to me: 1. It is true that *phobos* often means "horror" or "dread," but it also means "fear," and this seems to be the translation that best fits the definition by Aristotle himself in the *Rhetoric*: "*phobos* is the pain or disturbance resulting from the imagination of an imminent ill, either harmful or painful" (II, 5, 1382, a 21). 2. It is likewise true that Christian sensibility should not be allowed to interfere with our way of understanding the term *eleos*, but this does not prevent the "grief" of Hellenic *eleos* from referring also to a relationship between man and man: the painstaking investigation of W. Burkert has shown that in classical Greece the particular "grief" called *eleos* normally possessed an interindividual character. 3. The *ergon* of tragedy, what the latter by itself causes in the spectator, is not pleasure but catharsis; and in any event, the tragic *hêdonê*—which Pohlenz does not deny—must be understood in accordance with what Aristotle says of pleasure in the *Nicomachean Ethics*. 4. Tragic catharsis is, of course, a purgative process, but its essence is not confined to its momentary action; its most proper mission consists of setting the psychic life in order so that the impulses and rational appetites may remain subordinate to what is superior in the human soul, the intelligence; for Aristotle, man should not live "according to passion" (*kata pathos*), but "according to understanding" (*kata dianoian*). 5. Tragic catharsis, accordingly,

29. "Ueber die Anfänge der griechischen Poetik," *Nachrichten der Gött. Ges.*, 1920, and *Die griechische Tragödie* (Leipzig und Berlin, 1930); the latter was revised in its Göttingen edition in 1954.

also accomplishes a moral action. A Greek, a man in whose mind ethical sensibility and aesthetic sensibility, *to kalon* and *to agathon,* were always indissolubly joined together, would not have been able to conceive of the contrary. Even though the Greek theater was never a "sanatorium for moral cures," as Schadewaldt correctly states, tragedy had for the Hellenic people an unquestionable educative and ethical mission. The testimony of the *Frogs* of Aristophanes—I shall return to him later—is for Pohlenz wholly unexceptionable.

Thus so far the various opinions of those who have accepted the main body of Bernays' ideas consequently assert the analogy or identity between tragic and medicinal catharsis.[30] It seems not inaccurate to say that present-day philology sees a profound analogical relationship between attendance at a tragic drama and the process of an effective psychotherapeutic cure: in one and in the other the patient is psychosomatically calmed and relieved by what he hears and sees. But a close and synoptic examination of these opinions inevitably awakens in the mind of the reader—in mine, at least—a series of important objections. I see four as foremost among them:

1. The interpreters of Aristotelian thought on tragic catharsis usually limit themselves to considering the text of the definition of tragedy. Now it does not appear probable that this thought can be correctly understood without taking into account *all* that Aristotle says about the tragic spectacle and without methodically arranging the investigation within the frame of what tragedy was in its concrete historical reality and not merely, as Aristotle says, "in its essence." Schadewaldt lucidly warns of this need: "Now it would be necessary to examine," he says at the end of his study, "how the phrase here considered is *fulfilled* in the explanation of the parts of tragedy that follow it [in the text of the *Poetics*]. It is here and not in the *horos tês ousias* [in the "essential" definition of tragedy] . . . that Aristotle displays the total essence of the tragic"

---

30. I shall consider the thought of A. Lesky on tragedy, set forth by him in the first pages of his book *Die griechische Tragödie*, in the section of this chapter headed "The Tragic Action."

(p. 164). But the truth is that Schadewaldt does not carry out his own suggestion.

2. All the interpreters seem implicitly to accept Bernays' dilemma. *Katharsis* was for the Greeks, said Bernays, one of the following two things: *either* the expiation of a guilt by means of lustral rites, *or* the curing of a disease by purgative medicament; either purification or purgation. Tragic catharsis amounts, therewith, to purgation and purgation only. Even J. Croissant herself, who believes, as we know, that Aristotle must have taken that word from the religious vocabulary, ends by accepting the dilemma: Aristotle drew the term *katharsis* from the religious lexicon, she tells us, but he gave it a purely and exclusively medical content. Moreover, the psychosomatic reality of the catharsis to which the ritual enthusiasm leads—a thermal process, economy of black bile—would be in no way different from that which the physician promotes when he administers a purge; physiologically, all *katharseis* would be the same in the mind of the Stagirite. Let us admit this. Let us grant Bernays—why not?—that for a Greek of the fourth century the medical administration of a purge and the participation in a lustral or Dionysiac rite were things very different from one another. But can the careful and exacting historian ignore or underestimate the fact that medical catharsis had initially been understood in a religious sense by those who used it? Purgation with hellebore for the treatment of *mania* (*de diaeta,* I, 35, L. 6, 518) was in the fourth century a technical medical procedure; but Dioscorides informs us that hellebore was also called *melampodion,* because the physician-seer Melampus had cured the Dionysiac mania of the daughters of Proetus; and he adds that when people pulled it up to use it they were rejecting Apollo and Asclepius, the healing gods (*Mat. med.*, IV, 162). Something analogous must be said of squill, according to the investigations of E. Hirschfeld.[31] "Cathartic," O. Temkin rightly states, "is not *the* root of Greek medicine, but certainly one of its roots; a root that was not lopped off and discarded when scientific medicine gained pre-

31. "Studien zur Geschichte der Heilpflanzen," *Kyklos, 2,* 163.

eminence, but that continued fertile in metamorphosis. The particular quality of Hippocratic medicine could not be understood without it."[32] To purge a patient was also in a way to purify him, to free from excessive matter, to leave "pure," a portion of the divine *Physis*. This should not be forgotten when medical interpretation of any definition of the word *katharsis* is attempted.

3. Contrary to the interpretation of Dirlmeier—more or less openly admitted also by J. Croissant and P. Boyancé—tragic catharsis was not and could not be exclusively musical. The undoubted connection between the passage in the *Politics* and the definition of the *Poetics* indicates that Aristotle attributed a certain role to music in the production of tragic catharsis. To deny this is to deny the evidence. But that role had a secondary importance, since the power of tragedy, Aristotle says, holds good even without a public and without actors (*Poet.*, 6, 1450, b 19–20). In other words the *logos* of tragedy, what is said in it, is the principal agent of tragic catharsis.

Now present-day interpretations of the *pathêmatôn katharsis* consider above all the psychosomatic reality of the final effect of that catharsis: thermal and humoral processes, changes in the black bile, horripilation, tears. Let us grant all this as quite true; let us admit without reservation that this is what tragic catharsis was in the mind of Aristotle. But could it have been *only* that? Could Aristotle have failed to think of what happens within the psychosomatic reality of the spectator, in his *psychê* and in his *sôma*, from the time that the words of the tragedy struck his ear until his hair stood on end and his eyes shed tears? Between the ear and the skin of the listener, what happens to the tragic word? A reply must perforce be given to these questions if one wishes to understand fully what catharsis was for Aristotle.

4. The question of whether tragic catharsis did or did not

---

32. "Beiträge zur archaischen Medizin," *Kyklos, 3,* 101. E. Howald holds the same opinion ("Eine vorplatonische Kunsttheorie," *Hermes,* 54 (1919), and *Die griechische Tragödie,* Munich and Berlin, 1930) in respect to the unitary religious root—Pythagorean, he believes—of *katharsis*.

have a moral value to the eyes of its definer does not seem to have been formulated in its entirety. Along the lines of what one group and the other say, the defenders of the moralistic thesis are as right as the champions of the amoralistic thesis. Neither did the spectator attend the theater only to feel horror and to weep because this is secretly pleasing to the human soul, nor did he occupy his seat in the amphitheater in order to amend himself morally and become a better person. "The theater," Grillparzer rightly stated, "is not a correctional institution for rascals, nor an elementary school for the irresponsible." [33] But neither is it, I add, merely a place to shiver and weep pleasurably.[34] While awaiting the opportune moment to ask the question anew in a manner that I consider correct, two queries come to mind. Can one speak of the thought of the *Poetics* without taking into account the fact that its author was also the author of the *Ethics to Eudemus* and the *Nicomachean Ethics*? Can the problem of the effect of tragic catharsis upon the man who experiences it—more broadly, the problem of the psychological effect of tragedy—be formulated only in terms of "morality or pleasure"?

From my very modest position as a historian of the therapy of the word I shall attempt to arrive at an idea of tragic catharsis in which these four observations may find their corresponding reply. *Liceat experiri.*[35]

33. Quoted by A. Lesky, *Die griechische Tragödie*, p. 36.
34. Schadewaldt himself does not fail to recognize this. Aristotle, he says, did not think that the citizens of Athens went to the theater during the Dionysiac festivals because of having felt one day that there had gradually accumulated in them a too intense inclination to timorousness and emotionality, or because they noted themselves to be more than usually prone to explosions of wrath or fits of hatred, envy, pride, or desire for authority, to return to their homes relieved and calm. This is not what Aristotle considers essential in his definition of tragedy (pp. 156–57).
35. Such an attempt would be idle if, as Wilamowitz holds (*Einleitung in die griechische Tragödie*, 3d ed. Berlin, 1921, 110) it were not allowable to make use of that "inestimable treasure" of the *Poetics* in which tragic catharsis is mentioned. Wilamowitz writes: "Neither did Aeschylus seek to produce a cathartic effect nor the Athenians ever expect it. Perhaps the philosopher may have observed keenly and subtly the effect that a tragedy had upon the public or on himself

III. Some few years ago, in *Estudios de Historia de la Medicina y Antropología médica* (Madrid, 1943), I took the liberty of presenting a conception of tragic catharsis from a twofold point of view: the *logos* of tragedy and the most dependably valid theses of Bernays' interpretation. The *katharsis* of which Aristotle speaks to us must have been above all a "verbal catharsis *ex auditu*" comparable under changed circumstances to that which the orator in his audience and the psychotherapist in his patient can produce with words. Having read more widely since then (the foregoing pages well show how much ink has kept flowing in these last fifteen years) I shall set forth my thought, arranging it in several successive sections.

Attic Tragedy and Greek Life

The interpretation of Aristotelian *katharsis* must have as its point of departure a fundamental fact: the essentially religious character of Greek tragedy from Thespis to the creations of the last tragic writers. Even when at times tragedy lost the profoundly sacral accent that it had in the venerable days of Aeschylus, it always retained its essential bond with the religious traditions of the Hellenic people. "Divine service, part of the religious worship of the Greek State . . . the most perfect form attained by Dionysiac ecstasy," as Pohlenz defines it.[36] On the final page of *The Birth of Tragedy,* Nietzsche puts these words in the mouth of an Athenian: "Follow me to the tragedy, and let us sacrifice together in the temple of both di-

---

in his solitary reading, but such an effect was unknown to the poets and to the public." In my opinion the argument of Wilamowitz is not conclusive. Perhaps the Athenians may not have called the effect of tragedy *katharsis*, but the important thing is that tragedy produced in the spectator a well-determined effect, and that Aristotle applies this term to it. Of what does the phenomenon that Aristotle wished to call *katharsis* in his definition of tragedy properly consist? What did the philosopher propose to say with this expression, perhaps never before used in the same sense? This is our problem.

36. *Die griechische Tragödie,* p. 9.

vinities!"—that is to say, to Dionysus and Apollo.[37] With less poetic language and more positivistic philosophy, the anti-Nietzschean Wilamowitz must think the same: a Greek tragedy, his definition reads, is "a fragment of the heroic legend, complete in itself, treated by a poet in lofty style for a chorus of Attic citizens and two or three actors to stage in the shrine of Dionysus as an integral part of the public worship."[38] From the point of view of its form, tragedy was accordingly the Attic configuration of the primitive orgiastic and ecstatic dramatic performances of the worship of Dionysus; and from the point of view of its sense, as Zubiri has remarked, the pathetic version of Greek *Sophia*.

This profound religious character of tragedy—accentuated, if possible, by the heroic and traditional nature of the fables placed on the stage—confers upon the tragic author a special significance in the life of the Greek *polis*. The poet becomes the religious educator of his own people. In the dialogue that Aristophanes has Aeschylus and Euripides hold in the *Frogs*, the former asks: "Why should we admire a poet?" and Euripides' reply states: "For his intelligence and his admonishments and because we make men in the cities better" (*Frogs*, 1007–09). The bond between tragedy and the *polis* is at this point as clearly expressed as the educative role of the writer of tragedy. "For the younger children the educator is the school master, for youths the poet," Aeschylus later says in that same comedy (1054–55). The tragic poet, on the basis of the religious tradition of his people, making use of it moreover, educates the Athenians morally and religiously; the good art of the fable, the beauty of language and pageantry were but external notes—extremely important, but external—of the sublime function that the tragedy performed among the Hellenes. The Greek tragedic writer like the Christian preacher[39] expresses the religious and historical conscience of his contempo-

37. Despite his passionate musical "Dionysism," Nietzsche never went so far as to forget the Apollonian element—logical, verbal—of the Attic tragedy.
38. p. 108.
39. The comparison is Pohlenz's, p. 17.

raries in literary form; and at the same time, in carrying out his educative task, orients and governs with his work the attitude of the common man to his tradition and gods. The tragic author, in short, was for the Greeks an interpreter of their spiritual situation, a guardian of their destiny and helmsman of their behavior.[40] With which I do not of course mean to say that the Athenian stage was a pulpit or a house of moral correction.

Now comes the problem. In order to interpret Aristotelian *katharsis* adequately, should the characteristic educative quality of the Greek tragedy be taken into account? Such a procedure would not be allowable if Aristotle was blind, as Pohlenz thinks, to the real historical and social significance of tragedy. But is it true that the Aristotelian conception of the tragic poem does not go beyond being an aesthetic and hedonistic speculation? Pohlenz declares that a foreigner from Stagira, a man who was neither a citizen nor an Athenian, could not be

40. Up to Dirlmeier and Schadewaldt the opinion of philosophers in this respect has been very much in agreement. Wilamowitz expressly recognizes the educative and edifying function of the Greek tragic poem, even though he prefers to attribute it to its generic quality as a poem (p. 110). The passage from Jaeger reads in Highet's translation (3 vols., 2d ed. 1945, New York), *1*, 239: "That was the basis of its educational force, a force at once moral, religious and purely human" (*Paideia, 1,* 257). Nestle for his part writes that the tragedy "offered the possibility of showing the power of the divinity even over the fate of active and suffering man, and of making the cultal religiosity of the Athenian citizenry more lucid and profound, more intimate and enlightened" (*Vom Mythos zum Logos,* p. 169).

Schadewaldt defends his attitude by saying that the doctrine of Aristophanes in the *Frogs* is but a "Sophistic theory" foreign to the feeling of the Greek people, and that Aristotle is as opposed to it as he is to the well-known hostility of Plato to tragedy (p. 165). But Pohlenz replies that persons and authors not at all Sophistic also acknowledged that theory (Plato, *Ion,* 541b; Xenophon, *Convivium,* 4, 6), and the Sophists, for their part, were still Hellenes. The three great tragic writers, writes A. Lesky, "speak to the Athenians in the theater of Dionysus, and impelled by a sacred duty (Aeschylus and Sophocles) or with deep confidence in the power of the *logos* (Euripides) try to impart to them their knowledge about gods and men" (*Die griechische Tragödie,* p. 37). Lesky also reminds us that Homer was always a main subject in the education of Greek youths.

the "authentic expositor of Attic tragedy," and so it is that Aristotle "does not devote a single word to telling us that tragedy played a role in divine service and in the world of the heroes, nor does he even inform us that it was performed in the festivals of the *polis,* or that the tragic poet spoke to his people as its delegate." Was the author of the *Poetics* nothing but a sterile and formal preceptor?

It is poor procedure, no doubt, to discuss an author on the basis of what he does not say, and an even more serious matter to fail to adhere to what he really tried to do and say. With his *Poetics* Aristotle did not attempt to be a historian in the manner of Herodotus and Thucydides; very plainly he tried to be a propounder of the *technê poiêtikê,* and this he makes clear without beating about the bush at the beginning of his little treatise: "We shall speak of the poetic art in itself and of its species, of the essential function of each one of the latter, of how to compose the fable if one wishes the poetic composition to be beautiful" (1447, a 8–10). If this were not enough, his definition (*horos*) of tragedy is limited specifically in its reference to the "essence" (*ousia*) of the tragic poem (1449, b 23). The *logos* of the definition "sets the bounds of" essences —*horos* means precisely "limit" (*Top.,* I, 5, 101, b 39)—it does not describe appearances nor events. This and nothing else Aristotle tried to do, and we already know that it was not his custom to use words other than those necessary in each case. The Aristotelian concept of tragedy could not be and was not alien to the historical and religious life of the Athenians, even though the philosopher was a "foreigner from Stagira." That connection must not be sought in the essential words of a definition, but rather through the sense that the different concepts that Aristotle employs in his technical view of the tragic poem had for him.

Take, for example, the concept of pleasure or enjoyment (*hêdonê*). At least six times the *Poetics* refers to the characteristic pleasure of the tragedy: artistic limitation is a cause of pleasure (1448, b 18); pleasure characteristic of the tragedy does not consist in the good coming out well and the bad badly, nor in the two becoming reconciled to one another (1453, a 36); the tragic poet must seek the pleasure given by terror and compassion aroused through imitation (1453, b 10–12); tragedy, being a single whole, as is a living being, causes the pleasure proper to it (1459, a 21); the wonderful is a source of pleasure (1460, a 18); the tragic poem produces a specific pleasure (1462, b 13). There can be no doubt that the most proper and immediate purpose of tragedy is a particular *hêdonê*, an enjoyment specifically characterized by the features indicated in notes in the preceding passages; tragic *katharsis* is no more than a process aimed at producing in the spectator, in his soul and body, that particular enjoyment. Here Schadewaldt is completely correct.

Must we conclude then that Aristotle is proposing to us a hedonistic conception of tragedy? Of course. But under the condition that that *hêdonê* be understood exactly as Aristotle understood it, and not as we understand it when we speak or read the words "hedonist" and "hedonistic." Pleasure, *hêdonê*, is, the *Rhetoric* says, "a certain movement of the soul, and a total and perceptible return toward the natural state" (I, 11, 1369, b 33–34). Now a man can move in many ways toward what is natural to him, and so there exist for him many different types of pleasure. Among the several that the *Rhetoric* enumerates, the pleasures of marveling, struggling, or imitating appear to be the closest to the *hêdonê* of tragedy. But the *Nicomachean Ethics* also devotes itself to defining and describing human pleasure. Here the intellectual exactitude is greater. Pleasure is not a movement, nor is it a cause; it is a whole that does not increase with duration (X, 3, 1174, b 10, and 1174, a 17–19); pleasure consists in the unhindered activity of the habits that belong to the nature of the one who possesses them and exercises them (VII, 13, 1153, a 14–15); or, more precisely, in the perfection of that activity, even when the pleasure does not perfect the activity as an habitual form but as an end superadded to the form, just as the beauty of the body is added to the full development of youth (X, 4, 1174, b 31–33). All living beings, men or animals, endowed with sensibility desire pleasure in a certain sense. It is true that not all aspire to the same pleasure, but pleasure is that to which all aspire; for all beings, Aristotle concludes, have by nature something divine (VII, 14, 1153, b 32). This being the case, what can the pleasure most characteristic of man be? The Artistotelian reply is well known: that pleasure is happiness (*eudaimonia*): and although human happiness may demand material and external possessions (I, 9; VII, 14; and *Polit.*, 1331, b 41), the pleasure most suitable to it and at the same time most divine (X, 7, 1177, a 16–17, and 1177, b 30–31) is that which corresponds to the activity of thought. Among all natural realities man is, for Aristotle, a being doubly divine, if it may be meaningfully so put, and in accordance with this quality of his the pleasures of his particular nature acquire specific consistency and characteristic disposition.

What has been said indicates that in man's life there must be as many species of pleasure as there are activities; each pleasure in fact is paired with the activity that it perfects (X, 5, 1175, a 30). There are then dianoetic pleasures or those pertaining to thought, and somatic pleasures or those belonging to the body. These latter are more violent and more common, therefore the name of pleasure seems to have passed over to them as by inheritance (VII, 14, 1153, b 33), at least in the language of the common folk. Why are physical pleasures and delights more coveted as a rule than the others? According to Aristotle, for two chief reasons: firstly, because physical pleasure always has an opposing displeasure or distress (*lypê*) that may come to be excessive—when this occurs the physical pleasure to whose nature the power to expel the displeasure belongs is desired as one desires a medicament; secondly, because the pleasures of the body, on account of their intensity and even their violence, are pursued by men who cannot find delight in other joys. This occurs above all among the young (young men, Aristotle says, are like men intoxicated) and among the melancholy, who because of their humoral crasis live as though gnawed by a sort of anxiety and always need some medication or, in its absence, some physical pleasure sufficiently intense to serve as an expellant or repressive medication (VII, 15, 1154, b 11).

Within this doctrine, what can be said of the pleasure proper to tragedy? We know that in its production imitation (*Poet.*, 1148, b 18, and 1453, b 12), the marvelous (1460, a 18), terror, and sorrow-laden compassion (1453, b 12) have a part. Hence it is a pleasure at one and the same time dianoetic and somatic that accompanies the activity of following and vicariously living what is occurring on the stage; thus, acting as a medicament, and desired as such, it expels the displeasure caused by the excess of tragic emotions. Utilizing the compact vocabulary of the *Nicomachean Ethics* one can say that the tragic spectacle is at the same time pleasurable by nature and by chance (VII, 15, 1154, b 16–17). Pleasurable "by nature" (*physei*) is that which calls forth the most natural and characteristic activity of the subject who experiences the pleasure: in this case, thought. Pleasurable "by chance" (*kata symbêbêkos*) is that which produces pleasure as a medicament, because the therapy, Aristotle explains, is pleasurable inasmuch as it takes place through an activity of what is still sound in the organism: the "pleasurable by chance" in this case would be the psychosomatic state that the comprehension of the tragedy elicits.[41] The pleasure proper to the tragic spectacle—an end superadded to the activity that it accompanies—is in a way divine for two different reasons: because the all-seeing gods always intervene in the course of tragic action even though they may not be seen on the stage (*Poet.*, 1454, b 6), and because this pleasure belongs to the nature of the subject who experiences it, in this case, that of the doubly divine being that we call man. Now let it be said whether the Aristotelian conception of tragedy was or was not characteristic of the Hellenic mentality, and whether it corresponded to what tragedy was for the Greek people.

Another statement of Pohlenz, according to which Aristotle must not have been able to understand the sense of Dionysiac

---

41. It is certain that for Aristotle tragic pleasure would be more intense in individuals of melancholy temperament.

religiosity, seems equally unacceptable to me. I shall limit myself to setting down a few lines from W. Jaeger: "The seriousness with which the *Nicomachean Ethics* deals with enthusiasm, the high esteem for divination, for *tychê* [fortune] and for the instinctive, insofar as such instinctiveness rests upon a divine inspiration and not upon a natural inclination, in a word, the emphasis that Aristotle places on the irrational, is on the same plane as that idea of *peri philosophias,* according to which the irrational and clairvoyant forces of the soul constitute one of the two sources of the belief in God." [42] To demonstrate this, it is not even necessary to appeal to the youthful writings of Aristotle. In the *Nicomachean Ethics* the philosopher again tells us that the "good fortune" of the truly fortunate man has a "divine cause" (*theia aitia*) (X, 10, 1179, b 22), and in the *Poetics* itself he expressly highlights the specific efficacy of "mania" and "ecstasy" for the creation of the poem (1455, a 32–35). Moreover, among the literary ancestors of tragedy Aristotle cites the dithyramb, a song typical of the Dionysiac worship. And the deliberate appeal to the term *katharsis* in order to designate the pyschological action of tragedy—does it not perhaps expose the aim of arousing in the mind of the Greek listener an image to which the ceremonies of the worship of Dionysus belonged as much as did medical purges? The literal text of the *Politics* (1341, a 21–22) does not permit this to be doubted.

Or it may be that our idea of tragic catharsis—more precisely: our judgment in respect to what Aristotle was thinking in speaking of it—must very well take into account the religious and educative character that tragedy had for the Greeks of the fifth and fourth centuries and the religious as well as the medical emphasis that an ancient Hellene, whether physician, philosopher, poet, or simple citizen, never failed to perceive in the meaning of the word *katharsis.* More concisely, tragedy and its cathartic action had an essential connection with the beliefs of Hellenic man, both in his concrete reality and in the mind of Aristotle.

42. W. Jaeger, *Aristoteles* (Berlin, 1923), p. 251.

The Tragic Situation

In this title two concentric circles of meaning must be distinguished. The inner circle concerns the "tragic situation" in the strict sense: that in which the hero of the tragedy is vitally involved. The outer circle surrounding it has to do with the particular quality of the historical periods to whose content belong the living existence of the tragic and the creation of literary plays really and truly worthy of the name of tragedies. To avoid confusion, I shall call this second circle "tragic occasion". Let us examine in turn the "tragic situation" and the "tragic occasion," and let us attempt to see whether the *Poetics* of Aristotle has any relation to these questions.

The problem of the tragic has acquired in the past several decades a very active currency, especially, and not by chance, in the area of Germanic culture. As in so many other things, the fine historical flair of Max Scheler very early caught the scent of the renewed currency of the theme (*Ueber das Tragische*, 1914). Since that time zealous speculation about it has not ceased.[43] Is it possible to strike a balance of all that has been thought? In an excellent essay [44] of wide scope A. Lesky has tried to reduce the "essence of the tragic" to the six follow-

---

43. Here is a selection of titles: M. Scheler, "Ueber das Tragische," *Die weissen Blätter*, 1914, p. 758; J. Geffcken, *Der Begriff des Tragischen in der Antike* (Berlin, 1930); O. Walzel, "Vom Wesen des Tragischen," *Euphorion*, 34 (1933), 1; Th. Haecker, *Schöpfer und Schöpfung* (Leipzig, 1934); J. Bernhardt, *De profundis* (Leipzig, 1939); E. Bacmeister, *Die Tragödie ohne Schuld und Sühne* (Wolfshagen-Scharbautz, 1940); J. Sellmair, *Der Mensch in der Tragik* (Krailing vor München, 1941); F. Sengle, "Vom Absoluten in der Tragödie," *Dtsch. Vierteljahrsschr.*, 20 (1942), 265; W. Rasch, "Tragik und Tragödie," *Dtsch. Vierteljahrschr.*, 21 (1943), 287; A. Weber, *Das Tragische und die Geschichte* (Hamburg, 1943); H. Bogner, *Der tragische Gegensatz* (Heidelberg, 1947); K. Jaspers, *Von der Wahrheit* (Munich, 1947); H. J. Baden, *Das Tragische* (Berlin, 1948); H. Weinstock and K. von Fritz, *op. cit.* And why not cite as well Heidegger's work and the literary production of French existentialism? *Tragische Existenz* is the title of a work by A. Delp commented on in *Sein und Zeit*.

44. The chapter "Zum Problem des Tragischen," in *Die griechische Tragödie*, pp. 11–45.

ing features: 1. The dignity of the subject. For the "fall" of the tragic hero to be moving, his personal situation in the context of human destinies must be lofty. Aristotle was referring to "dignity" such as this when he spoke of the "valiant" or "lofty action" of tragedy. 2. The possibility of relating the conflict to the personal world of the individual who considers it as a spectator. 3. The clear awareness of the hero in regard to the situation in which he finds himself. Without it the situation on stage may be piteous but not tragic. 4. The irreconcilable character of the tension or opposition to which the hero finds himself led. The pessimism and the despair of modern man have accentuated to the greatest possible degree the inexorability of this definitive quality of the tragic. But is the tragic opposition among the gods, between divinity and man, or between two halves of the same man always irresoluble and irreconcilable? This does not appear to be so sure a thing. No one will refuse to grant the *Oresteia* its quality as a tragic trilogy because Orestes comes out well in it. Lesky solves the question by distinguishing the "exclusively tragic view of the world" (that belonging to those who assert the total irreconcilability of the tragic tension) and the "exclusively tragic conflict" (that of an opposition not reconcilable in itself, but capable of solution in a superhuman order of reality which is the object of faith).[45] In a really Christian world the first is not possible because human existence and the cosmos have for the Christian a sense that transcends rational order; but the second certainly is possible, and thus, in accord with Bernhardt and against Haecker, the possibility of a true "Christian tragedy" can be understood. 5. The existence of a "tragic flaw" not morally ascribable. The hero of a tragedy commits an error, of which, in a mysterious fashion, the tragic action is an objective and unavoidable consequence; but he does not therefore cease to be subjectively innocent (K. von Fritz). 6. The possibility of discussing

---

45. Lesky adds yet a third possibility, represented by what he calls "tragic situation," in which, without the lessening of its genuine "tragic" quality, a favorable solution is still possible. Such would be the situation of Orestes after he had slain Clytemnestra and Aegisthus.

whether the tragic event has any meaning for us or if, on the contrary, it is totally lacking. Is the course of tragedy absurd or not? Hebbel, Scheler, and many of the present-day "existentialists" decidedly maintain that it is. Sengle, Jaspers, and Lesky himself think that there is always an "absolute" and "transcendent" order in which the tragic action can have a reasonable sense, an order transcending the human as such and all of history in the most arduous and extreme conflicts, and transcending only what I have above called the "tragic occasion" in less serious cases. "His downfall," writes Lesky, speaking of the tragic hero, "is inevitable but it does not lack meaning. His time is not yet ripe for the value for which he fights and falls; but his sacrifice leaves the way free for a better future."

These words bring us into the second of the two circles defined above: the "tragic occasion." To human existence there belongs a radical impoverishment as regards its own destiny. It is what Dilthey once called "the permanent corruptibility of our life" and what Ortega has before his eyes when he says that the life of man is a "problem" and a "shipwreck." To be a man on earth is to live in a way that is essentially deficient, problematical, and precarious, to which what one believes and knows give a certain degree of security, never a total security (Ortega). "However powerful and godlike man may be," Sengle writes, "he dwells in the shadows of twilight, however wisely constituted and disposed a human creature may be he ends as a victim of destruction, however pure the path of a hero may be he always falls into guilt." [46]

But the feeling of his own deficiency that man possesses gains special vigor and prominence in definite historical situations, precisely those in which tragedy is born and lives as a literary genre. They are times in which man, without having lost the support of faith that his existence finds in the bosom of his people's religious and historical traditions, begins to part with them, eager for personal autonomy yet insecure in the unbound administration of his own existence and even fearful of it. More concisely, they are periods in which a crisis in the

46. Sengle, p. 265.

basic beliefs of a historical community has begun to take place. Audacity toward the holy and fear of the holy then become intermingled in souls in a confused and anguishing way.

Tragedy sets forth a literary picture of this situation through an individual and outstanding human destiny. Here is presented as a drama the life of a man who moves and struggles in the border area of human existence, that zone in which the possibilities of being a man are most grave and threatening. The tragic poet depicts on the stage the conflict of a noble and valiant person who seeks to live in himself—Orestes in Argos, Antigone in Thebes—and who yet does not know how and cannot do it, perhaps because that which he seeks is not and will never be possible in his world, or perhaps, in a more radical way, because it is not humanly possible. One might say that the tragic hero *lives* in his world, but he *is* not of his world. Thus his adventure ends in tragedy, in a painful and pitiable conflict. The outcome of the tragic action is then the return of the man to the belief that, wounded and living at one and the same time, still continues to give support to his soul and to his people: a return that necessarily must pass through suffering or through death—this latter in the case of true tragedy—because the hero has gone beyond the bounds reached by his own sufficiency as a man of his world, or perhaps as a mere man. Only by suffering and dying can he who has transcended the limits within which he was able to guide his own steps by himself be reconciled to reality. We find ourselves left, accordingly, with this moderate conclusion: tragedy stages the life of a man in a *new, unforeseen,* and *extremely grave* situation of his own existence; the tragic poet educates the spectator by showing him what that man can do and does in such a situation. The educative action of tragedy is, accordingly, moral—nothing in the life of man can be amoral—but on a much more profound plane than that to which this word usually refers.[47]

This is ultimately the reason why tragedy as a literary genre has existed in three historical situations only: Greece of the

---

47. Jaeger has been wise enough to perceive well that incipient break between religious faith and the autonomy of man which lurks deep

fifth century (crisis in the beliefs of the Greek world), modern Europe (crisis of the beliefs of the Middle Ages, secularization of life), and the present-day Western world (crisis of beliefs proper to the secularized world, progressive optimism and faith in pure reason: Kafka, Sartre, Faulkner, Miller).[48] And that too is the cause of the troubling coincidence of tragedy and philosophical originality in the history of culture. Genuine philosophy indeed seems to be an inseparable historic companion of suffering, even though the personal life of the creative philosophers may be easy and placid. "How much this people —the Greeks—must have suffered to be so beautiful!" wrote Nietzsche; and he also could have written: to be so wise. The endeavor to "abolish from the essence of tragedy the element of reason, of the *logos*, of wisdom, on account of its musical and ecstatic component" (Nietzsche) is, therefore, radically erroneous even though it may not be wholly unfounded. The immortal words of Aeschylus: *pathei mathos*, "through suffering knowledge," could be the motto of all Greek tragedy (Nestle).[49] In the "historical occasion" of tragedy, communal

---

within the Greek tragedy. He alludes to the "unburdening of fate" upon the head of the tragic hero and to the vicarious experience of that unburdening on the part of the author and the spectator of tragedy and writes: "If that shared experience of the unburdening of fate that Solon once compared to a storm was to be resisted, the greatest strength of man's spirit was necessary on his part; and against fear and pity—the immediate psychological effects of the vicariously shared situation— that vicarious experience demanded faith in a meaning of life as a last reserve" (*Paideia, 1,* 268). The same in H. Weinstock, *Die Tragödie, and Sophokles* (Berlin, 1947). On the constituent "morality" of human acts—at times in the form of "im-morality"—see the *Ética* of J. L. L. Aranguren (Madrid, 1958).

48. Problems pile up. What meaning does the tragedy have in the life of peoples, and individual men, who continue rooted in their ancient faith? How is a Christian tragedy possible? Was there really "tragedy" in the theater of Calderón? In Lope's drama are *El castigo sin venganza* and *El caballero de Olmedo* true tragedies? Was *La Celestina* one?

49. "Suffering," Jaeger comments, "entails the force of knowledge. This fact belongs to the most ancient folk wisdom. The epic does not make use of it as a dominant poetic motif. In Aeschylus it acquires a more profound and central significance. The 'know thyself' of the Delphic god constitutes an intermediate stage, which demands the knowledge of

and sustaining belief, as I have said above, is at one and the same time wounded and living. More wounded in some men, more living in others, it is the pressing argument that makes possible the dramatic and existential arrangement of the tragic event.

It would be useless to seek in Aristotle a theory of the tragic: Aristotle does not give one. It would be foolish on the other hand to demand of an ancient author that he view the history of man with a historical conscience similar to ours. But if one sharpens his sight in reading the *Poetics,* evidence of an intellectual attitude toward tragedy very much in keeping with what has been said will be revealed. Aristotle clearly states the need for the dramatic action to be lofty and noble; he emphasizes vigorously the guilt-free quality of the error (*hamartia*) into which the tragic hero falls; he alludes expressly to the "undeserved" (*anaxios*) character of the suffering that that hero undergoes (1453, a 5–16); and he considers Euripides the "most tragic" (*tragikôtatos*) of all the poets because in his tragedies the number of fatal outcomes is greatest —Euripides, the tragic writer of the period in which the favorable or conciliatory solution of the Greek tragic conflict was most difficult. The author of the *Poetics* was not a simple preceptor. He was a philosopher—*et pour cause!*—and he knew how to scrutinize the tremendously deep historical and human problem of tragedy.

The Tragic Action

Tragic catharsis could not be understood were it forgotten that tragedy is above all the imitation on the stage of a *human action.* The *Poetics* is permeated throughout by this conceptual theme: the most important part of tragedy is its plot or argument (*mythos*), precisely because the plot imitates or repre-

---

the limits of the human, as Pindar constantly teaches with devout Apollonian piety. . . . But this does not exhaust the Aeschylean conception of the *phronein,* of tragic knowledge by the force of suffering" (*Paideia,* 1, 273).

sents *praxis*, an *action* of men (1448, a 23; 1448, a 27; 1449, b 24; 1450, a 15 ff). The fundamental difference between tragedy and epic would be rooted in the character of the former, at once active and performable: all the tragic characters are on stage, Aristotle expressly says, *prattontas kai energountas*, "acting and in action" (1448, a 23). The plot, and hence the action, is literally the soul of tragedy.

The relation between the character of the tragic drama and the property of human life represented by it is set forth with great vigor in the following passage:

> The most important of these parts—the six constitutive of tragedy—is the linking of the actions, because tragedy is not an imitation of men but of an action and a life; happiness and misfortune [50] are in the action of man, and the goal is an action, not a quality. For men are such as they are according to their character, but are happy or wretched according to their acts. The players do not act to imitate characters, but they receive their characters by reason of their actions; so that human acts and the plot are the goal of tragedy, and in all things the goal is most important. (1450, a 15–23)

The idea that the happiness, misfortune, and goodness of a man should refer to his activity as a man and not to a quality or a habit is very characteristic of Aristotle.[51] His definition of goodness in the *Nicomachean Ethics* is well known: "The activity of the soul according to the best and most perfect virtue" (I, 6, 1098, a 18).

In summary: tragedy represents the destiny of a man in action; hence his happiness or misfortune and the possibility that the soul of the spectator may vicariously experience one or the other. Inasmuch as the *telos* or proper and immediate end of tragedy is the imitation of a human action, the specific

50. I adhere to the text proposed by Gudeman as opposed to that of Hardy and others.
51. *Nicomachean Ethics*, I, 6–7, 1098, a 16 and b 21; *ibid.*, X, 2, 1173, a 14; *ibid.*, X, 6, 1176, a 34; *Phys.*, II, 6, 197, b 4; *Polit.*, VII, 3, 1325, a 32.

hêdonê or enjoyment of the tragic drama—let it be remembered that pleasure is the perfection of an unhindered natural activity—must consist in the auspicious or fatal disposition of that action, imaginatively and emotionally participated in by the public, within the possibilities of the existence of the tragic character and of the spectator himself.

The Inner Arrangement of the Tragic Action

This human action in which tragedy has its "soul" is not what is commonly called "pure action," it is not the action of a mere "activist." It is arranged and articulated by means of the word and discourse, by means of the *logos*, hence "logically." Together with the dialectical or convincing *logos* of the *Organon* and the rhetorical or persuasive *logos* of the *Rhetoric* it is now necessary to posit a new type, the tragic or cathartic *logos* of the *Poetics*. However great the role of the Dionysiac and orgiastic element may have been in the production of the tragic effect (lyric poems, choric songs), the word in which the action was expressed played a much greater part: tragedy springs more *aus dem Geiste des Logos* than *aus dem Geiste der Musik*, despite the genius of Nietzsche.

No one could evaluate the expressive and verbal—"logical" —element of tragedy better than the inventor of logic. In the very definition of tragedy, and as soon as he has pointed out the intimately "active" character of tragic imitation, Aristotle prescribes that such action is to be expressed "in well seasoned language." It was the merit of Aeschylus, he says elsewhere, "to lower the importance of the chorus and give the first place to the discourse of dialogue" (1449, a 6–17). The tragic action is inseparable from language; so much so that when Aristotle enumerates and defines the six constitutive parts of tragedy, he expressly considers elocution or *lexis* as "the fourth of those pertaining to language" (1450, b 13). The other three are the plot or action, the thought or "ability to say what is fitting to the situation," and characterization, which is made real and manifest in the course of action that the speaker adopts or avoids. Hence the *Poetics* can say that "the plot should be so constructed that even without seeing it acted out the one who hears it will be seized by trembling and compassion" (1453, b 3). Tragic action can cause its proper effect upon the soul of the hearer even when it is reduced to pure discourse or *logos*. Auditory sensations are those which leave the greatest impression on man, Theophrastus will subsequently say (frag. 91 W).

The interpretation of tragic catharsis must not lose sight of this structured, orderly arrangement that the word imprints upon the action of tragedy.[52] If the tragic poem imitates in a poetic and pathetic manner an extreme vicissitude of human destiny, thanks to the *logos* the fulfillment of two essential qualities of the drama is possible: the suitable, orderly arrangement of that collision of man with his unconquerable destiny and the correct understanding of the conflict on the part of the spectator. He who participates in Dionysiac orgy *becomes part* of it, while the performance of the tragic poem is viewed. A theatrical performance and viewing are called in Greek *theôria*, and the latter is possible in the theater and in the life of the philosopher only thanks to the *logos*. What was concurrent, direct participation in Bacchic enthusiasm becomes in the theater imitative contemplation. Tragedy was the brilliant result of that taming of the Dionysiac bull by the Attic word.

THE POSSIBILITY OF TRAGIC ACTION

The human action that the Attic tragedy imitates, represents, or proposes through language has this singular prop-

---

52. It can now be understood, contrary to what Dirlmeier asserts, that the *katharsis* named in the *Politics* is not identical to the *katharsis* of the *Poetics*. In the former music is fundamentally the active element; in the latter, together with *melopoiia*, the *logos* as well. It is true that the *logos* also has a musical component, the intonation of what is said (Book III of the *Rhetoric*); but it is necessary to agree that in the effect of the word the "what" of the speech—what is said with it—is considerably more important than its "how."

erty: it could happen to the spectator himself as a man and, more immediately, as a Greek.

Hardly had the Hellenes set themselves to reflect on the poetic phenomenon than they realized with the greatest clarity the constitutive character in it of the personal participation of the individual who hears or reads the poem. Gorgias speaks of poetry and tells us: "I judge poetry in its totality as speech with meter. He who hears it finds himself assailed by awe-inspired trembling, tearful affliction and weeping that takes pleasure in its grief, and in the face of joyful events, matters and persons foreign to him, he feels in his soul his own passion as a result of the word" (EH, 9). It is evident that Gorgias is thinking primarily of tragedy. A passage from his works more expressly referring to the tragic poem has an analogous sense: "Tragedy . . . is a deceit in which the one who deceives is more just than the one who does not deceive, and the one deceived wiser than the one who is not deceived" (frag. 23 Diels). Only if that "deceit" or "fiction" which is tragedy constitutes for the spectator a real possibility of his own life, only then can the one deceived be prudent and his illusion just.

This essential quality of tragic action does not escape the keen eye of Aristotle. When in a famous passage he wishes to show that poetry is more philosophical than history, he begins by contrasting the character of their respective narratives: "History tells the events that have happened, poetry those that could happen . . . Poetry narrates the general and history the particular. The general consists of the fact that it befits a given quality to speak or act in a certain way, according to verisimilitude and necessity . . . and the particular, of what an Alcibiades has done or has undergone" (1451, b 5–11). Therefore if the character in the tragedy represents credibly the *general* quality of being a man, Greek or Athenian, the Athenian spectator will always feel more or less represented in the action of the tragedy. What occurs on the stage to the tragic character can also occur in the life of the spectator. The insistent argumentation of Aristotle about the possibility of the tragic action in itself (1451, b 15) and the frequency with which he warns in regard to the "verisimilitude" of the plot point very directly to the imaginative possibility of the tragic event in the fate of the spectator.

The production of tragic catharsis demands that the spectator of tragedy vicariously experience its plot as a possibility in the course of his own life. This possibility may be vaguely felt or clearly and distinctly understood by him; it can be a formless feeling or an articulate piece of information. Aristotle calls *philanthrôpon* (1452 b 38; 1453, a 2; 1456, a 21) the feeling of community and solidarity with which the spectator vicariously experiences the misfortune of the hero; and according to the *Nicomachean Ethics* (VIII, 1, 1155, a 20) that *philanthrôpon* is the human equivalent of the affective bond existing among animals of the same species. Accordingly, in the bosom of the two tragic passions, fear and compassion, and in the bond of friendship linking the spectator to the hero there is always a more or less express and clear preconceptual framework: the awareness that the tragic action viewed *is possible* in the life of him who views it. If this were not so the spectacle of tragedy would be no more than pastime or archaeology.

Qualities and Course of Tragic Action

Tragic action must be valiant and thrilling. Otherwise there would be no tragedy; the spectator could not experience fear and compassion. "The imitation," Aristotle notes, "has as its object not only a complete action, but also incidents that arouse fear and pity" (1452, a 1). But neither would there be tragedy if the action were not *unexpected* and *surprising* or *marvellous* to the one viewing it. The Aristotelian idea of *katharsis* could not be understood without bearing very well in mind these lines of the *Poetics:* "Since such passions—fear and pity—are aroused particularly *when the incidents occur against our expectation,* even though they issue from one another [53] [the marvellous is an effective element of tragedy];

---

53. That is to say, even though there is a "credible and necessary" connection among them.

for the marvellous will have a greater effect than [if the incidents seem to arise] by chance and fortune, since among the incidents due to fortune we judge the most marvellous to be those that appear, so to speak, intended" (1452, a 3–7). Hence the causing of fear and pity, and of their consequent catharsis, demands that the development of the action take place against the expectations of the spectator. The incidents must follow one another with "credibility and necessity,"[54] even though this necessity or *ananké* of human behavior— what man does because it fits his natural character—may not be equivalent to the necessary "providence" of the movements of the universe. Finally, the impression of "surprise" or "wonder" that the thread of the tragedy must arouse is achieved when the incidents, beside being unforeseen, seem to be intentional. Tragic actions appear to us as such when to the unexpectedness of their course are joined threat and enticement, two of the possible directions into which "the unforeseen" can be diversified.

This essential impression of the tragic event in the mind of the spectator becomes evident in the "change of fortune" (*metabolé* or *metabasis*) that the hero must experience on stage, and even more so when that change of fortune takes the form of a "reversal" (*peripeteia*) or turn of the tragic action in a direction opposite to the one that the foresight of the spectator was expecting. The reversal carries to its highest point the feeling of surprise that the change of fortune necessarily arouses and must be considered, according to Aristotle himself, as a kind of irony of fate (*Hist. anim.*, VIII, 2, 590, b 13–15).

Let us briefly review what occurs in the tragic spectacle. On the stage a human action both extreme and terrible is simulated. The speech of the characters, skillfully and poetically composed by the author, accomplishes a twofold mission: it expresses that action in an orderly way and enables the spectator to experience it vicariously as his own. The tragic plot is broken up into several incidents, linked in their course by the

54. The "character" of the persons of the drama gives credibility and necessity to the series of diverse acts within the tragic plot.

double bond of credibility and necessity. But the internal necessity of the tragic action does not carry with it a sure predictability of the various incidents composing it. On the contrary the emergence of the tragic effect demands that some one of these incidents be unforeseen and surprising to the spectator, but for all that without failing to seem freely and intentionally decided by the character. The incident on stage then acquires the quality of the marvellous.

At this point, accordingly, as a result of a change of fortune, and even more when the latter takes the form of a reversal, the spectator arrives at a state of mind characterized at the emotional level by fear and pity (or by dread and grief, as Schadewaldt proposes to say) and at the intellectual level—if you will, at a "logical" level—by disorientation, a tense and confused disorientation. Things are not happening on the stage and in the mind of the one viewing them in agreement with the unpremeditated expectations that he has been forming throughout the drama. In all of it there is a curious mixture of fiction and truth: of fiction, because the tragic action merely imitates reality in a poetic form, and of truth because the spectator, carried away by the action that he sees and hears, lives it as if it were really happening in his own life. To this subtle mixture of illusion and reality Gorgias was referring in the passage quoted previously.

How can the spectator get out of that strange situation into which the change of fortune and the reversal have thrust him? He has only one path available to him: to clear up the predicament, to set in order expressly and articulately the confusion caused by the downfall of all his disappointed expectations. This illumination of the tragic action after the surprise of the reversal is the *anagnôrisis* or *recognition:* "the transition from ignorance to the knowledge that leads to friendship or enmity among those destined to happiness or misfortune," according to the definition of Aristotle (1452, a 29–32). Thanks to the *anagnôrisis* the spectator escapes from his momentary confusion and "realizes" what is happening on the stage and therefore in his own life.

Aristotle distinguishes between simple and complex plots or, as the old preceptors used to say, "implexed." When the change of fortune takes place without reversal or *anagnôrisis* it is said that the action is simple. The unforeseeability and the surprise of tragic action then remain limited to pure *metabasis*. When the *metabasis* entails reversal and *anagnôrisis* the tragedy has a complex plot. These are the tragedies that the *Poetics* considers most perfect.

The statement that there exist *anagnôrisis* not preceded by a reversal is implicit in the foregoing paragraphs. To be precise, the idea that Aristotle has of *anagnôrisis* is so broad that it extends to the recognition of inanimate beings (1452, a 34). Any recognition of anything unknown up to a given moment, by virtue of which the tragic action becomes more clear and undisguised, for the character and for the spectator, is an *anagnôrisis* in the mind of Aristotle. "The most beautiful *anagnôrisis*," he tells us, "is that which is joined to a reversal" (1453, a 33, and 1454, b 28); "the best thing is for one to perform the action without being aware of it [without realizing whom it will affect], but with *anagnôrisis* after performing it" (1454, a 2); "the best recognition," he concludes, "is that which is derived from the facts themselves" and not from discovering schemes, external signs, scars, and necklaces (1455, a 18 ff). Reversal, thoughtlessness of the character in respect to the final consequence of his acts, and support of the recognition by the facts themselves are, in short, the notes that define the good dramatic quality of *anagnôrisis*.

I need not explain and comment here on the five types of recognition that Aristotle distinguishes nor the considerations of the philosopher on the greater or lesser poetic suitability of the several possible reversals. It is important, on the other hand, to emphasize the extraordinary attention that the *Poetics* devotes to *anagnôrisis*. This means that a situation of surprise and confused ignorance—it is attained by a simple change of fortune or through reversal—is fundamental to the production of the tragic effect in the mind of the spectator. Even the best-known traditional myths were able to cause astonishment. "It is not absolutely necessary," says Aristotle, "to adhere to the traditional plots that serve as a basis for tragedies. It would even be a ridiculous concern, for the things known (fables, myths or legends) are known to a small number, and yet they entertain all" (1451, b 15).[55] Let us be wise enough to understand in all its significance this singular importance of recognition.

The Affective Aspect of the Mental State

A valiant, terrible, vicariously experienced, and marvellous human act must immediately produce in the spectator a singular state of mind. Aristotle does not exhaust his vocabulary in the endeavor to define it. With exemplary conceptual and stylistic self-restraint he prunes from his prose all verbal luxuriance and leaves us these words as his entire description: "by means of pity and fear"—or of grief and dread, if Schadewaldt's version be accepted—"the tragic poem carries out the purgation of such passions." The state of mind proper to tragedy is described only with two positive notes: fear and pity. This is not saying too much, but perhaps it may be saying enough.

The yoking of fear and pity is far from being new in Greek literature. Gorgias and Plato used it, perhaps with a descriptive purpose like that of Aristotle. But the existence of such historical precedents does not exclude the Aristotelian enumeration from referring to an immediate psychological experience.

What in fact does tragedy represent? Let us have Aristotle

55. Gudeman (p. 163) has tried to diminish the importance of the "ignorance" in which the course of the tragic action places the spectator. Aristotle's expression here cited must have been merely an "epigrammatic subtlety," especially when the poet explained in the prologue of the tragedy the content of the tragic action. But Gudeman's argument is not conclusive. One may have seen *King Lear* five times and be moved on the fifth occasion as much or more than on the first. The prologue itself would rather fill the function of an apéritif for the tragic emotion. I think that Aristotle would not be displeased by this dietetic or medicinal conception of the action of the prologue.

himself tell us. "It is the case of a man who, without being superlatively outstanding in virtue and justice, falls into misfortune; not because of his badness and perversity, but because of some error of his" (1453, a 7). On the tragic stage a man of noble and lofty soul is beheld (1448, a 17), but not so eminently virtuous that he cannot be viewed by the spectator as his peer and fellow and even as representing his own life. On that man misfortune obstinately, cruelly, and undeservedly falls. What state of mind is possible to the spectator who really vicariously experiences that fate as his own? He will feel for the moment fear and trembling. "Fear [*phobos*]," the *Rhetoric* tells us, "is the pain or perturbation that results from the mental image of an imminent ill, whether harmful or painful . . . and this if it seems not distant but imminent" (II, 5, 1382, a 21-25). The orator who wishes to instill fear into the minds of his audience is then instructed. It will be best, Aristotle suggests, to sway them "by telling them that they are in a position for something to befall them because others too, greater than they, have suffered, and by showing them that others like them are suffering or have suffered" (II, 5, 1383, a 9-11). These passages of the *Rhetoric*, so generically conceived by their author, can be applied quite justly to the understanding of the tragic effect. Tragedy too suggests in an immediate fashion the imagination of an approaching, destructive, and imminent ill because before the public a man is suffering whom the audience can, after all, consider as its peer. What passion but fear can then be dominant in its state of mind?

Not only fear, but compassionate grief as well. Pity (*eleos*), Aristotle tells us, is

> a certain pain as a result of a misfortune, appearing grave and painful, in someone who does not deserve it, which a person, or someone near to him, could expect to suffer himself, and this when it appears imminent; for it is clearly necessary that the person who is going to feel pity

should be in such a situation as to be able to believe that either he himself or someone near to him is going to suffer, and an ill such as has been indicated in the definition, or a like or almost equal one. (II, 8, 1385, b 13–19)

The repeated mention that Aristotle makes of pity throughout the *Poetics* has here, accordingly, a double meaning. On the one hand, it completes the description of the tragic emotion in the person of the spectator: a fear such as tragedy arouses must be accompanied by compassionate grief.[56] On the other hand, the Aristotelian conception of pity fully affirms one of my previous statements: when the spectator of tragedy experiences pity he feels confusedly or perceives with emphatic clarity that the grievous and terrible action is possible in his own destiny. The Aristotelian idea of tragic catharsis could not be independent of the author's thoughts on pity and fear.

How are the two tragic passions produced in the spectator? "Fear and pity can arise," we are told, "from the stage presentation and also from the very sequence of incidents, which latter is preferable and the mark of a better poet" (1453, b 1). The action itself is what should produce fear and pity, not the use of tricks and artifices extrinsic to the thread of the tragic plot. This shows us that the plot which best arouses in the public the mental state proper to tragedy (1452, a 39) by means of reversal and *anagnôrisis* will always be complex; and this is so because it is then that the tragic event becomes most unexpected and marvellous to the eyes of the character and of the spectator. "These passions," Aristotle unhesitatingly asserts, "arise particularly when the incidents occur against our expectation" (1452, a 3), that is, when they are simultaneously credible and surprising.

And if the tragic action were not enough by itself, there is the chorus. "The chorus," Wilamowitz has written, "is for the

---

56. It is probable however that for Aristotle the simultaneous presentation of the two tragic emotions was not indispensable. Gudeman (p. 163) nicely observes that the words *phobos* and *eleos* are not always connected by the conjunction *kai*.

The Power of the Word in Aristotle

Attic tragedy not only an active character, it is also the spokesman for the feelings and thoughts that the author proposes to elicit through the action." [57] The chorus represents the human group that most directly shares with the hero the terrible vicissitudes of his fate. Its members are, among other things, a class of spectators closer to the tragic action and more immediately affected by its marvellous incidents; and their singular situation makes them at the same time intermediaries of the tragic effect and orienters of its concrete expression in the minds of the audience. The choragus was in a way a popularizer of the lofty and difficult doctrine that the action of the tragedy contained in respect to the destiny of man—of man in general and of Grecian man.

The Genesis and Structure of Tragic Catharsis

Perhaps we are now in a position to understand in its entirety the genesis and structure of tragic catharsis exactly as Aristotle must have understood it.

To this end let us try to reconstruct in its real dynamics the situation of the spectators of a tragic performance in fifth and fourth century Athens. During the Dionysiac festivals, and as part of the worship by the *polis* of the god of Bacchic enthusiasm, fertility, and wine, the Athenian would attend the performance of a tragedy. From the steps of the theater he saw taking place on stage not only a portion of the heroic legend poetically wrought by the author but also a possibility more or less close to his own fate. Some men, Greeks like him, based upon the same mythical and religious tradition, thrust into the same historic destiny, and believing in the same gods, are weaving before his eyes the fabric of a valiant and grievous event. They move within the zone of human life that seemed most difficult and extreme to the ancient Greek: that in which

---

57. *Die griechische Tragödie*, 2, 145. See also, in respect to the function of the chorus, W. Jaeger, *Paideia, 1* ("The drama of Aeschylus"), and the article "Hypokrites," by A. Lesky in the volume honoring Paoli (Florence, 1955).

man feels impelled and at the same time torn by a secret tension between fate and freedom. The perpetual difficulty and the grave danger in which the tragic hero finds himself overwhelm the mind of the spectator with vague disquietude. Everything on stage is beautiful, surprising, and terrible. Fear and pity take possession of the soul. The spectator fears for the hero, but in the hero he fears for himself; with his own grief he sympathizes with the misfortune of another, and in this sense the misfortune *is* to a degree his, but he also feels the unhappiness of the hero inasmuch as that unhappiness *could be* wholly his. The change of fortune breeds terror, grief, and confusion; the reversal brings spiritual tension to the highest degree; the intensity of the emotion thus keeps rising to a peak, that is to say, until the *anagnórisis* resolves the terrified and grievous initial confusion into clearer and more distinct fear and pity. Thanks to the *anagnórisis* the spectator knows and recognizes what really is occurring on stage and therefore is his own possible fate; and he knows it in a specific way, arranged in orderly fashion, in fair words, in credible actions, and in precise sensory images. The original confusion of life is transformed into order, a sorrowful or happy order, depending upon the denouement of the tragic action, but at length crystal clear. Only because the *anagnórisis* permits it can there be a denouement, fatal or fortunate, in the course of the tragedy. Only by virtue of the recognition do the truth, the inner coherence and the meaning of the plot—a superhuman meaning, almost always—become evident in the mind of the spectator. The *anagnórisis* represents, in short, the triumph of that deep demand for expression and clarification of the human destiny—a figurative, verbal expression and clarification—that in the face of every possible purely musical and Dionysiac interpretation beats deep within the breast of Attic tragedy.

The *Poetics* calls this "resolution" of the affective state of the spectator *katharsis*. Why did Aristotle choose this name, at one and the same time religious and medical? I think because of the double reason implicit in that double meaning: because of what the tragedy still had of Dionysiac worship—"Aristotle was thinking of the time when the theater had not yet separated from worship," J. Croissant correctly writes [58]—and because of what there was of psychosomatic and medicinal "purgation" in the affective "resolution" following the *anagnôrisis*. In any case, it seems necessary to distinguish four main stages in the structure of tragic catharsis.

In the first place its *religious-moral stage*. Let us not forget that tragedy was part of the worship of Dionysus. The music that accompanied the tragic performance, aside from the merely acoustic or tonal effect that it might exert because of the character of its melody (there is music that excites and music that soothes), necessarily had to arouse in the public memories and emotions of religious character. But more deeply and clearly than the music the content of the tragic action itself placed the spectator face to face with a deep religious and moral problem ultimately referable to the conflict between traditional faith and the noble will to independence of the hero. Error, virtue, bravery, and misfortune were disturbingly entwined in his life under the gaze of the gods, and almost always by their decision. Whether the spectator likes it or not, there his own religious and moral beliefs are at stake. Solon had said that whoever possesses as much as he can possess reaches out his hand to take twice as much. The sin of *hybris* or excess is a constant temptation for the soul of man. "But what in Solon was merely a reflection on the impossibility of man's limitless appetite ever feeling satisfied," Jaeger comments, "in Aeschylus is transformed into the *pathos* of a bond between demonic seduction and the overpowering of man by its brilliance, who follows it without resistance on a road to the abyss." Hence the ambivalent moral conscience of the tragic hero—obscurely mingled in it are the feeling of his own justice and the feeling of his own guilt—and below the surface the need for expiation that is piercing his soul. Let us not forget that tragedy, as a historical phenomenon, is inseparable from the *guilt culture* that the Archaic Age was for the Greek

58. p. 58.

people. The denouement of the tragedy, a final metabasis toward happiness or toward misfortune (*Poet.*, 1455, b 28) would prove to be the adverse or happy result of that longing for expiation.

Aristotle says that "by means of imitation man gets his first knowledge" (*Poet.*, 1448, b 7). Tragedy, a poetic imitation of traditional legend, also gives knowledge, "knowledge at the price of pain," according to the formula of Aeschylus. From Thespis to Euripides, each tragedy is a bold step by Athenian man toward the conquest of hitherto untried possibilities of existence, dangerous and, in their beginning at least, terribly confused. The brilliant poetic undertaking of the great tragic writers constituted a trial of the Greek spirit, a counterpart of that which the philosophers from Thales to Socrates began at the same time in respect to intellectual knowledge of *physis* and of being. A verse of *Prometheus Bound* expresses with special vigor this Athenian task of learning to be a man—a Greek man—through tragedy: "This I know," says the chorus to Prometheus, "because I have seen your annihilating fate" (553). Never has the chorus represented more profoundly the spectator of the tragic poem.

But knowing, even though it be through pain and death, cleanses the soul of confusion and puts man more in possession of himself. And thus, not only in the tragic emotion of the spectator, in his fear and in his pity, is there an essential religious and moral moment, it is also present in the catharsis of those passions and in the pleasure that necessarily accompanies the latter. The fatal or fortunate outcome of the tragedy reorders existence with respect to what is most central and decisive in its structure, namely its relation to divinity. And when life itself or its fictional representation on the stage reveals that reality, "a very few words are sufficient," Sengle writes, "to make the meaning of the world, the Absolute that is above all disharmonies, shine anew with purity." Which, I add, is also a cathartic process.

To the tragic state of mind and the catharsis into which it is resolved belongs in the second place a dianoetic or logical point. The knowledge of which I have spoken is not an ineffable illumination; it is above all a psychological process of verbal expression. Through the *anagnôrisis* the spectator learns to express in an orderly and satisfactory way what is happening on the stage and what is happening in his soul; he passes therefore from inarticulate confusion to articulate knowledge. I shall not repeat here all that has already been said. But I cannot resist the temptation to copy a few significant lines from Nietzsche:

> At the sight of the myth that was unfolding before him the spectator felt himself exalted to a sort of omniscience, as though the visual power of his eyes did not remain at the mere surface and were able to penetrate into the innermost secrets of things; as if now, thanks to music, he were beholding before him, perceptible to his senses, the out-pourings of the will, the struggle of motives and the swollen stream of the passions, like an abundance of lines and figures in a lively motion, and could thereby plunge into the most delicate secrets of the unconscious stirrings.[59]

If this lofty paragraph be divested of its Nietzschean garb, if the influence of music be assigned its proper place, it will not be difficult to reduce it to essentially what I, in interpreting Aristotle, have said in respect to the clarifying power of the *anagnôrisis*. Certainly the "catharsis of the passions" was also an intellectual or dianoetic process.

Easier to see, and even more important in the Aristotelian definition of tragedy, is the *pathetic or affective point* of the tragic state of mind and of the catharsis resolving it. The plot with its religious and moral gravity, the cruel fate of the tragic hero, the dignity of the language, the music, the beauty of the pageantry—"the beautiful is but the first degree of the terrible," Rilke has written (*Eleg. Duino*, I, 2-3)—all conspired to produce the two tragic passions and the feeling of vital community (*philanthrôpon*) that served both as a basis. That fear, pity, and the feeling of vital community had, as Schadewaldt

59. *Die Geburt der Tragödie*, section 22 (ed. Kröner), *1*, 173.

asserts, the quality of "elemental psychosomatic emotions" is something that cannot be doubted; that the tragic "terror" of the Athenians was an emotion merely comparable to the thrilling psychosomatic anguish of a vegetative neurosis is however a questionable matter. If the classification of human activities into "higher" and "lower" be admitted by way of orientation, it is necessary to recognize that the tragic passions were aroused by appeals very much "higher" than coenesthetic sensibility or by the simple visual perception of a terrifying object. All that I have been saying up to this point shows this clearly. And the same can be maintained in respect to the catharsis of such passions. Tragic catharsis was no doubt the "purging" or elimination of emotions that did not exist in the soul before the viewing of the tragedy, and it occurred when the emotional tension reached its peak. But the impulse unshackling the cathartic process did not come to the spectator "from below"—from his viscera and his humors I mean to say, even though the tragic state of mind might affect both—but "from above," from the dianoetic enlightenment elicited by the *logos* of the poem. The words of the tragic poem, insofar as they concerned the beliefs of the spectator, stirred up and promoted passions; insofar as they were expressive of a terrible, threatening, and surprising fate, the well-composed climax of those words made the emotional tension extremely great; insofar as they determined an enlightening knowledge, they swept confusion out of the soul and induced catharsis. Not only in philosophy; in tragedy as well the *logos* is superior to *éthos* and *pathos*.[60] To assert the contrary would have been a grave insult to any of the three great tragic authors.

Finally comes the *somatic or medicinal point* of tragic catharsis. The words of the poem entered the ear of the spectator and reached his mind, but they did not remain there; they had also an effect upon his humors and hair. The three cathartic processes to which Aristotle refers in different places in his works—the enthusiastic or musical, the medicinal or purga-

60. On the significance of the *logos* in ancient philosophy, see E. Grassi, *Vom Vorrang des Logos* (Munich, 1939).

tive, and the tragic—must have coincided in their somatic or terminal reality. The painstaking and excellent philological investigation of Jeanne Croissant and Hellmut Flashar has shown us in great detail the physiological thought of Aristotle concerning the thermal, humoral, and symptomatic aspect of the two tragic passions (coldness and moisture of the excretions, changes in the black bile, horripilation, shivering, palpitation of the heart, weeping) as well as the mechanism of cathartic purgation, even though with respect to the latter theme neither of the two authors has considered that the agent of tragic catharsis is not a material purgative, nor even a melody, but rather that airy, invisible, material, and immaterial reality that we call the "word"—a fact quite forgotten by subtle contemporary philology, at times more inclined to pursue purges than to esteem language.

From this somatic and medicinal point of view tragic catharsis would be the return of the crasis of the spectator to a more balanced and natural, hence more healthy and pleasurable, humoral and thermal state than the one immediately preceding the cathartic process. But neither should it be forgotten that, even though the consideration of the interpreter be restricted to the physical aspect of purgation, the Hellenic idea of medicinal catharsis was not independent of the religious thought of the Greek people. The link between the one and the other was twofold: the general attribution of a divine character to the *physis* and the real meaning of the word *katharsis*, a sense from which a deep religious ingredient was never absent in the mind of the Greeks. "Purgation" was also "purification," and more so when it was a question of leaving a portion of the *physis* "pure." We have already seen how hellebore was *at one and the same time* a purge and an agent of purification, *katharmos*.

Now we can understand in a properly complete fashion what the characteristic pleasure of tragedy, the *oikeia hêdonê* of the tragic poem, was for Aristotle. "Each one is brought pleasure by what befits his nature," says the *Politics* (1342, a 25). Accordingly, tragic catharsis was pleasurable because it was suitable to the *whole* nature of man. This of course was so because it produced a thermal and humoral purging of the crasis, especially intense in the melancholy, by means of which the body of the spectator might return to a state more in harmony with his nature, more *kata physin*. But this element of *hêdonê* was merely resultant or terminal. Previous to it and determining its genesis were and had to be those pertaining to the good order of the soul, both of affective character (having to do with the *thymos*) and of intellective nature (concerning the *dianoia*), for the Divinity is thought and man "does not ultimately live as a man except insofar as he has within him something divine" (*Nicomachean Ethics*, X, 8, 1177, b 31). Pleasure, I shall once more repeat, is the perfection of an unhindered natural activity, superadded or crowning perfection (*epiginomenon*), just as the physical beauty of the youth is added to the fullness of his growth. The activity on which tragic *hêdonê* bestows pleasure and perfection is an existential transition—dianoetic, affective, and physical at one and the same time—from confusion and disorder to well-ordered enlightenment. Aristotle says that there is not only activity in movement, but in the freedom to move as well. Hence, passing from the realm of appearance to the realm of essences, the tragic pleasure would be that belonging to the human activity of knowing oneself better and disposing more freely and consciously of one's own destiny.[61]

61. The tragedy grants the spectator the possibility of exercising his freedom in a new and wished-for area of his own life. The end is foreseeable. Practicing again and again the enterprise of living for and by himself, the Greek loses his original faith; the possibility of writing original and "living" tragedies ends in Athens and the creative life of Greece dies out. The tragedies of Euripides "bring the spectator onto the stage," as Nietzsche says; the believing and tormented hero of ancient times becomes the enlightened, reasoning man, almost indifferent to the traditional faith of the second half of the fifth century and the first half of the fourth. Thereupon the tragic cycle in Greece closes, even though subsequently in the fourth century so many tragedies are written. The living experience of a tragic *katharsis* kept fading by degrees until it became a mere archaeological curiosity. It is possible that Aristotle may have been a witness of that final period of catharsis. It appears certain in any case that his mind was able to perceive all the deep

Is not the pleasurable and well-ordered state of mind produced by tragedy the same that the "fair speeches" of Socrates were to arouse in the soul of young Charmides, and to which Plato wished to give the already illustrious name of *sôphrosynê*? A finely intuitive conclusion of Menéndez Pelayo on the "purification of the affections," as it used to be said, or "purgation," as we have preferred to say since Bernays, so states:

> The purification of the affections, once it has been stripped of scholastic ostentation and the numberless subtleties and cavillings in which commentators have entangled it, proves to be nothing but the re-establishment of *sôphrosynê*, the tempering and calming of the passions so divinely praised in the Socratic dialogues. The difference is merely in the fact that Aristotle expects such effects from art itself and from dramatic imitation, demanding of the artistically idealized passion a remedy for the real passion that each spectator bears in his breast.[62]

Menéndez Pelayo's intuition is indeed subtle and accurate, but it merely poses the problem. The difficulty will begin when an attempt is made to explain how that "real passion" has come about in the breast of the spectator and how the "idealized passion" can be an effective remedy for it.

Comparison of Opinions

I think that my interpretation of tragic catharsis includes and places in a more comprehensive, unified order those of Jeanne Croissant, Schadewaldt, and Flashar. And on the other hand it also gives an adequate account of those others where it is preferred to consider the metaphysical aspect of *katharsis*,

---

meaning of the cathartic process in which the "ingenuous" beholding of a tragedy used to end. Some generations later tragic catharsis will be a memory, a subject for conversation or for instruction for the use of "snobs," rhetoricians, philologists, and aesthetes. Or of writers of the history of medicine, as is now the case.

62. *Historia de las ideas estéticas* (Santander, 1940), *1*, 74.

such as Untersteiner's, or to emphasize primarily its ethical and moral quality, such as Volkmann-Schluck's, Schottländer's, and Stark's, or to highlight its intimate religious force, such as Weinstock's and Sengle's.

I venture to say as much of the historical and psychoanalytical conception of Pohlenz. Aristotle proposed to save the tragedy from the damning judgment that Plato had cast upon it. Among the several effects of the tragic poem upon the spectator, Plato saw very much in the foreground the stirring up of irrational emotions. Poetry would strengthen the irrational elements of the soul at the expense of the reason, and this makes it worthy of condemnation in the eyes of Plato. "A man who had conceived of tragedy as pyschagogy," Pohlenz comments, "was one who could least impugn the fact that it had irrational effects and produced pleasure by the satisfaction of a psychic *dynamis* thirsty for tears and lamentation. But if Aristotle wished to save tragedy, he had to show that that satisfaction does not lead to strengthening the irrational in man at the cost of reason. The famous doctrine of catharsis serves this end." And later he adds:

> Plato rejected tragedy because it strengthens the irrational part of the soul by the stirring up of the emotions. Aristotle replies *psychoanalytically* that if this strengthening takes place, it is by reason of a violent repression. With much more vigor than his master he recognizes the irrational impulses as natural and useful and therefore considers their appetite for satisfaction as natural. He holds their excess, however, to be harmful and sees in the vicarious experiencing of another's pain the purgative therapy that affords a harmless discharge to the excess and reduces the emotions to their just measure. He who purifies himself is certainly the same man, and it is he also who finds relief under that feeling of pleasure. There for Aristotle is the source of tragic fruition. But the habitual language of physicians offered the occasion to speak of the purging of the emotions, and in that sense the term is

used in the famous definition of tragedy, a definition of which *katharsis*, as the principal factor, is the emphatic conclusion.[63]

With *katharsis* the soul would recover good order among its various parts.

Aristotle, in short, attributes to the word—to the express and communicative *logos*—a threefold power. When the human word is dialectical reasoning it convinces; when it is rhetorical discourse it persuades; when it is a tragic poem it purges and purifies. The foregoing pages have shown the essential relation that verbal persuasion and catharsis have to medicine and the curing of human illness. But this connection will be made still more evident by viewing the thought of Aristotle within the constant Greek concern for the psychological action of the word. Such is the main objective of the "Conclusion" which follows.

63. *Die griechische Tragödie*, pp. 529–531.

Conclusion

With the death of Aristotle original speculation on the psychological action of the human word, and hence on its curative power, comes to an end. I do not think that the Stoic doctrine of the *logos prophorikos* and moderation of the passions adds anything really substantial to what Plato and Aristotle had already said in regard to verbal psychagogy.[1] Only with Christianity—within which the divine person who "became flesh" will be called *Logos*, "Word"—will a new possibility begin for verbal psychotherapy; but this possibility, only incipient in Gregory of Nyssa, Basil of Cappadocia, and Clement of Alexandria, will take centuries to bear fruit, and its fruits will not always have a Christian appearance.[2] It seems then that this is the proper time to summarize the verbal psychotherapeutic legacy of classical Antiquity from a twofold point of view, historical and systematic.

I. In the Homeric epic it is already possible to collect data on the use of the word for curative purposes. Moreover a careful reading of the *Iliad* and the *Odyssey* reveals that the uttering of words on the occasion of human illness takes three forms radically different from one another: the prayer (*euchê*), the magic charm (*epaoidê*), and the suggestive or cheering speech (*terpnos logos*). The action of the latter must have had a purely and exclusively natural character.

But the social importance of the persuasive word is so great in post-Homeric Greece and its effect upon the man on whom

---

1. Professor W. Leibbrand and his pupils in Munich are studying with great perspicacity the psychopathology and psychiatry of the Stoic philosophers. Their investigations may make it necessary to rectify or to modify this negative judgment.
2. Again I refer the reader to my *Introducción histórica al estudio de la patología psicosomática*.

it acts is found to be so wonderful that poets and thinkers begin to call it metaphorically *epôdê,* charm, and *thelktêrion,* spell. As though he had been charmed or bewitched man changes his state under the influence of the persuasive word. It cannot be surprising that some (Gorgias, Antiphon) conceived the idea of applying it "technically" to the curing of certain maladies.

Plato also calls the effectively suggestive word *epôdê,* no longer as a simple metaphor or extrinsic analogy but as a literal or intrinsic analogy. Hence he finds himself obliged to explain the reason for that analogy. The suggestive word can be called a charm whenever it is a "beautiful speech" (*logos kalos*) and when as a result of being such it produces in the soul *sôphrosynê,* a beautiful, harmonious, and rightful ordering of all the ingredients of the psychic life: beliefs, feelings, impulses, knowledge, thoughts, and value judgments. This is achieved by reorganizing the contents of the soul around the axis of its active beliefs, or by eliciting in it new beliefs and persuasions more noble than the old. Such would be the proper function of "mythical" language as opposed to the convincing and inexorable efficacy of "dialectic" reasoning. And that reorganizing and enlightening process of the persuasive word receives from Plato the old and suggestive name of *katharsis.*

Now *sôphrosynê,* a virtue of the soul, is of medical importance from a twofold point of view: it produces beneficial somatic effects—so much so that without *sôphrosynê* complete health could not exist—and is a prior condition for the best and greatest efficacy of medicaments. Accordingly, the knowledge of a physician would not be "technically" complete if he were unable to produce *sôphrosynê* in the souls of his patients. Thereby the endeavors of Gorgias and Antiphon acquire intellectual justification and there arises, in a truly technical and rigorous form, the doctrine of verbal psychotherapy.

The Hippocratic physicians, the physicians continuing Hippocrates' work, were not wise enough to take up and make their own the legacy from Plato. It is true that they were acquainted with verbal psychotherapy, but they used it merely to win the confidence of the patient and to maintain in good tone his threatened spiritual "morale." The *technê* of the Hippocratics did not know how to become *dia tou logou technê,* a verbal art, though it could have done so. The "therapy of the word" —the technical knowledge and utilization of the *physis* proper to the human word or the *physiologia* of the *logos*—never came to have real existence in scientific traditional medicine.

Aristotle takes possession of the legacy of Plato, but in his own way. He will devote an entire treatise to the persuasive word, the *Rhetoric,* in the body of which it is not difficult to glimpse the possibility of "therapeutic oratory." And on the other hand he will distinguish in the *Poetics* a new manner of the word's action, the "cathartic." Plato had called the convincing and persuasive reorganization of the soul "catharsis": a convincing argument, he says on one occasion, is the chief and highest of the *katharseis* (*Sophist,* 230d). The Stagirite, in contrast, calls *katharsis* the purgation that certain words, those of the tragic poem, can produce in the whole reality of the human being. From the point of view of their effect on the one who hears them there are thus three distinct *logoi:* a dialectical or convincing *logos,* a second, rhetorical or persuasive, and a third tragic, purgative, or cathartic. The Aristotelian study of the persuasive *logos* is implicitly related to verbal psychotherapy; in contrast, the purgative or cathartic *logos* has in the work of the philosopher an essential and express relation to medicine. For Aristotle a physician who was able with his words to produce in certain patients psychological effects similar to those of the tragic poem would be therapeutically more effective and complete than the one who sees therapeutic practice as only a "mute art," in the manner of the Vergilian Iapix.

Did the Aristotelian physician Diocles of Carystus take up this lesson from Plato and Aristotle? Perhaps. Fragment 92 from Wellmann says: "Diocles considered friendly solace as a charm [*epaoidê*]. For it stops the flow of blood when the *pneuma* of the wounded man is attentive [in this case: when the attention of the mind of the wounded individual is great] and remains as if bound to the one who is speaking to him." [3] The sons of Autolycus also used an *epaoidê* to stanch the hemorrhage of Ulysses' wound. But Diocles is here not calling *epaoidê* a magic charm but, like Plato in the *Charmides,* the consoling and suggestive word of the physician. Psychotherapeutic *rapport* is very concisely and vigorously described in those two lines from Diocles. Whether or not the psychotherapeutic treatment to which the physician of Carystus refers is capable of such an intense hemostatic effect, is the intellectual heritage of Plato expressed in his words? Possibly. But the historian's conjecture can now go no further than to point out such a possibility.

Although Diocles had eyes to see the psychotherapeutic doctrine of Plato, medicine after the fourth century did not follow his path. When that medicine was scientific it ignored verbal psychotherapy; when it had recourse to the therapeutic use of the word it was not "scientific" medicine but magical and superstitious practice. The magic charm did not disappear from popular cures, nor even from many others that appeared to be above common superstition.[4] "If you tell me your ailment," Pleberio said to Melibea more than two thousand years after the *Odyssey,* "it will be cured at once, for there will be no lack of medicines, or servants to seek your health, whether it is in herbs or in stones or in words or hidden in the bodies of animals" (*La Celestina,* Act 15). And the vogue of the charm in folk medicine, as we all know, does not end with the publication of *La Celestina.*

II. Such, in its general features, is the adventure of the therapy of the word in classical Antiquity. Since history has not ceased to be *vitae magistra*—although in quite a different sense from that given by Cicero and the historical pragmatism

3. M. Wellmann, *Die Fragmente der sikelischen Aerzte* (Berlin, 1901).

4. I again refer the reader to the articles "Epode," by Pfister, and "Aberglaube," by Riess, in the *RE* of Pauly-Wissowa, and to the study, *Greek Medicine in its Relation to Religion and Magic,* by L. Edelstein.

of the Enlightenment to these words—let us try to consider systematically the lesson taught modern man by the brief history set forth in these pages.

For the production of psychological and therapeutic effects of any importance, the word, the Greeks tell us, must be "beautiful" (*logos kalos*). The human condition of the hearer and at times even his very imperfection demand this (Aristotle, *Rhet.*, III, 1, 1404, a 7–8) because good external embellishment of speech helps to persuade and for many is even the most efficacious element. Yet this demand for beauty pertains not only to the external and ornamental notes of speech, but also to its purity, propriety, good order, and above all to its adequacy.

Only when the word comes from a man of prestige and is accommodated to the character and the mood of the hearer, only then will it become fully efficacious. The prestige of the speaker is based on his natural qualities (a certain talent for pathetic eloquence, like that of actors: Aristotle, *Rhet.*, III, 1, 1404, a 15), his moral qualities (integrity, prudence), and his skills (mastery of the matter in question and of the art of speaking). More useful than anything to the speaker would be his prestige and knowledge if he is unfamiliar with what the hearer requests or needs on that occasion. This depends upon three distinct though closely interrelated psychological factors: the character or *êthos* (in which are fused nature, *physis,* and education, *paideia*), the condition or *diathesis* (to which the illness and its character in the case of curative oratory belong), and the occasion or *kairos* (the chance state of the hearer in the course of his life). Moreover, for the action of the word to attain its greatest efficacy—and psychotherapeutic treatment especially demands this—it is necessary that a particular relationship be established between the speaker and the hearer: the latter must have made a sort of "presentation" or *paraschesis* of his soul to the former (Plato) and must listen as though tied to him by the bond of attention (Diocles).

The necessary relationship between the speaker and the

hearer has now been established. The orator has now begun to speak. When will his speech be really apt? The reply of Plato and Aristotle coincides: when that speech is able to stir up passions (*pathê*) and beliefs (*pisteis*) in those who hear it. Now this disturbance can take place in two different ways. One is gentle, purely persuasive. By persuasively arousing new beliefs in the mind of the hearer, or by modifying with art and tact those in it that might already exist, the psychagogic word creates in that mind a new order, more "natural" and proper than the one existing prior to the speech, or corrects the disorder (*ametria*) from which the constitution of the psychic life may have been suffering. This is what Plato calls "catharsis of the soul"; it is the *Platonic verbal catharsis* or the simply persuasive catharsis.

But there is another and more violent way to stir up passions and beliefs which consists in exciting by the word a state of confusion and emotional tension and in bringing this state to a climax, to resolve it then abruptly by means of suitable and timely verbal expressions. The transition to the "new order" is now rapid and entails a considerably more active bodily participation than in the previous case. It is accordingly more pleasurable to the senses. Of this the process of *Aristotelian verbal catharsis* consists: "verbal catharsis" in the strong sense of this expression.

All this, as is evident, has a close relation to medicine. The bond that the Greeks saw between the action of the word and the curing of illness was threefold. The good order of the soul always has beneficial physical consequences, both in the state of health as well as in the state of illness. Moreover, that good psychic order would be a necessary condition to make best and most effective the curative action of drugs, diet, and surgery. And in the case of Aristotelian verbal catharsis the action of the word is so intense that it operates as though the speech itself were an actual medicament.

This, then, is the outline of verbal psychotherapy that the philosophers of Greece mapped out and the Greek physicians were not wise enough to take up and make their own. The philosophers did indeed believe in the curative action of the word and thought about it with more or less explicitness. Not even from this very particular point of view were they unfaithful to the potent verbal genius of Hellenic tradition; but neither did they fail to realize the limits of the transforming power of the word. On a previous page I have transcribed an old elegiac passage relative to this limitation. "If the sons of Asclepius had received from the gods the power to cure wickedness and perverseness," Theognis wrote, "what rich rewards they would receive! If reason were a thing that could be produced or instilled into man, never . . . would he whom wise speeches would have persuaded have become an evil man" (I, 431–36). A curious thing: two centuries later Aristotle will have recourse to that same poetic text when in the final chapter of the *Nicomachean Ethics* he seeks to show the need for coercive laws. The persuasive speeches that Theognis longs for, thinks Aristotle, are effective for the education of noble-spirited youths but are not able to attract the masses toward the good and the beautiful. The common folk do not obey a moral sense of honor but fear. "What speech could convert such men? It is not possible or it is very difficult to destroy with the word very deeply rooted habits" (X, 10, 1179, b 17). Man can be virtuous by nature when divinity so determines (*theia aitia*), but also by custom and by instruction. "But the word and doctrine do not have enough force for everyone, and the soul of the hearer must be cultivated by habit to love and to hate right-mindedly, as the earth is prepared to receive the seed. For no one who lives by passion will hear and understand the dissuasive word. In his case, how will it be possible to persuade him by words to be another? It can be said in general that the word is not sufficient against passion and that force is necessary. Nevertheless, there must somehow be a habit near to virtue, loving the beautiful and rejecting the ugly" (1179, b 25–31). Hence, Aristotle concludes, just law is unavoidable that "has coercive force and is at the same time a discourse that comes from practical understanding and the mind," from *phronêsis* and the *nous* (1180, a 22–23).

May not these words of Aristotle be transferable to medicine? Let it be recalled that in the view of the Hippocratics a correct treatment is equivalent to a "just law" (*de fract.*, 7, L. 3, 442). Accordingly, going "beyond Hippocrates" as Plato wished to do, let us interpret that expression after the manner of Aristotle. When the root that the illness has taken in the *physis* of the patient is intense and lasting, the word of the physician is not sufficient to cure. It is necessary then to associate with it "force" in the form of a medicament, diet, or surgical operation. But there can be no correct medical treatment, just as there is no just law, unless there exists and works in it, together with its "coercive" elements, a beautiful speech that emanates at one and the same time from practical understanding and from the mind. Classical Antiquity always says or is able to say something of value to the ear of the man who seeks its company with love. I venture to think that this old rule of Western culture has seen itself once more confirmed.

Index of Authors

Adrados, F. R., 51, 89
Aeschylus, 27, 33, 34, 37, 40, 42, 44, 51, 53, 58, 65, 66, 67, 68, 69, 70, 103, 203, 206, 216, 219, 232
Alcman, 64
Alcmeon of Crotona, 39, 81, 124, 132, 139, 142, 143
Allen, J. T., 66
Amman, J. C., xxiii
Anacreon, 64
Anaxagoras, 12, 48, 87, 142
Anaximander, 31
Anaximenes, 12
Antiphon, *97-105*, 106, 118, 126, 137, 139, 151, 163, 166, 173, 180, 241
Aranguren, J. L. L., 216
Araujo, M., 120, 184
Archilochus, 51, 72
Aristides Quintilian, 77
Aristophanes, 39, 59, 65, 102, 103, 205, 207
Aristotle, 14, 59, 61, 67, 73, 80, 101, 133, 138, 142, 144, 162, *171-239*, 240, 242, 244, 245, 246, 247
Aristoxenus, 78
Artelt, H., 17, 128
Ast, G. A. F., 100
Aulus Gellius, 46, 106

Bacmeister, L., 212
Baden, H. J., 212
Basil of Cappadocia, 240
Batteux, C., 185, 186
Bernays, J., 185, 186, 187, 188, 189, 190, 195, 199, 200, 201, 204, 237
Bernhardt, J., 212, 213

Bias of Priene, 89
Bidez, J., 83
Bignone, E., 83
Bogner, H., 212
Böhme, J., 9
Boissonade, J. F., 135
Botto, A., 3, 4, 5
Boyancé, P., 35, 39, 41, 42, 43, 49, 54, 58, 74, 76, 77, 108, 113, 120, 127, 130, 193, 202
Brendel, D. Adam, 7
Buchholz, E., 5
Buffière, F., 1, 10, 12
Bühler, K., 151
Burkert, W., 199
Burnet, J., 74, 83
Bywater, I., 189

Caelius Aurelianus, xxiii
Calderón de la Barca, 216
Castelvetro, L., 185
Censorinus, 81
Chantraine, P., 8
Chapelain, J., 185
Chion, 137
Cicero, 162, 243
Clearchus, 162
Clement of Alexandria, 56, 240
Clements, F. E., 8
Coglievina, B., 5, 7
Combarieu, J., 45, 78
Contenau, G., 26, 30
Corax, 67, 91, 172, 173
Corneille, P., 186
Cornford, F. M., 33, 74, 76
Croissant, J., *189-93*, 201, 202, 231, 235, 237

Daremberg, C., 5, 7, 142
Deichgräber, K., 101, 140, 145, 164

249

Index of Authors

Delatte, A., 76, 77, 83, 87, 107
Delp, A., 212
Democritus, 12, 77, 87, 90, 103, 105-07, 139, 142, 151
Deubner, L., 35
Diehl, E., 20, 51, 64, 89
Diels, H., 44, 73, 74, 77, 82, 83, 92, 98, 103, 104, 105, 106, 221
Diès, A., 92, 105, 119
Diller, H., 101, 140, 145
Diocles of Carystus, 171, 242, 243
Diodorus, 53
Diogenes of Apollonia, 12
Diogenes Laertius, 75, 76, 82, 85, 98
Dioscorides, 201
Dirlmeier, F., 193, 197, 206, 220
Dodds, E. R., 2, 6, 19, 32, 33, 36, 41, 42, 43, 74, 108, 113, 123, 127, 132, 135
Döring, A., 189
Dufour, M., 174
Dumézil, G., 75
Dumortier, J., 69

Ebert, M., 22, 25
Edelstein, E. J., 41
Edelstein, L., 40, 41, 46, 107, 120, 139, 140, 143, 164, 243
Eliade, M., 22, 42, 74, 75
Else, G., 149
Empedocles, 36, 43, 44, 82-86, 87, 90, 142
Englert, L., 42
Epictetus, 86
Epimenides, 35, 42, 74
Eunapius, 135
Eupolis, 63
Euripides, 35, 40, 48, 51, 52, 53, 63, 64, 65, 66, 67, 69, 70, 194, 205, 206, 217, 232, 236

Faulkner, W., 216
Fernández Galiano, 110
Ferrater Mora, 76
Festugière, A. J., 122, 127, 169
Finsler, G. A., 7
Flashar, H., 127, 181, 237, 278, 280

Fleischer, U., 139
Fredrich, C., 140
Frenkian, A. M., 9, 12
Freud, S., 83, 181
Friedrich, J. R., 5
Fritz, K. von, 188, 212, 213
Frölich, H. F., 5
Fuchs, R., 142

Galen, 3, 60, 179
Geffcken, J., 212
Gernet, L., 97
Gigon, O., 74
Glotz, G., 19
Goethe, W. von, 193, 197
Gomperz, H., 105
Gomperz, T., 96, 105
Gorgias, 63, 67, 82, 85, 88, 91-97, 98, 99, 100, 101, 102, 107, 118, 120, 126, 137, 139, 163, 164, 165, 166, 167, 172, 173, 188, 221, 224, 226, 241
Götze, Heinz, 80
Grassi, E., 234
Greene, W. C., 53
Gregory of Nyssa, 240
Grillparzer, F., 203
Gudeman, A., 185, 218, 226, 228
Gurlitt, W., 107
Guthrie, W. K. C., 43, 76
Guyton de Morveau, 3

Haecker, T., 212, 213
Hardy, J., 185, 218
Hebbel, C. F., 214
Heidegger, M., 177, 179, 212
Heim, Karl, 108
Heinimann, F., 88, 89, 97, 101, 104, 105, 177
Heraclides Ponticus, 75
Heraclitus, 80, 83, 86, 87, 142, 148
Heraclitus rhetor, 7, 10, 19
Hermogenes, 98
Herodicus of Leontini, 97
Herodicus of Selimbria, 139
Herodotus, 33, 34, 36, 38, 50, 64, 75, 207
Herrlich, S., 41
Herzog, R., 41, 139, 143

Index of Authors

Hesiod, 20, 33, 43, 61, 64, 79
Hippocrates, 9, 73, 77, 124, 132, *139-40*, 164, 170, 171, 241
Hirschfeld, E., 201
Höfler, A., 77
Hoffman, W. J., 78
Homer, *1-31*, 32, 34, 38, 42, 43, 55, 61, 63, 79, 197, 206
Howald, E., 71, 72, 73, 188, 202
Hundt, J., 36

Iamblicus, 75, 78, 79, 81, 82, 187
Ibycus, 64, 66
Isaeus, 190
Isocrates, 93, 173
Italie, G., 66

Jaeger, W., 5, 9, 33, 73, 74, 83, 105, 140, 143, 146, 149, 155, 161, 164, 175, 206, 211, 215, 216, 229, 231
Jaspers, K., 212, 214
Jayne, W. A., 41
Joel, H., 97

Kafka, F., 216
Kerény, K., 41, 76
Kindermann, H., 71
Kleingünter, A., 41
Koller, H., 188
Kommerell, M., 193, 196
Körner, O., 3, 5, 7, 18
Kranz, W., 12, 33, 74, 80, 83, 98

Laberthonnière, L., 28
Leibbrand, W., 98, 240
Lesky, A., 5, 50, 193, 200, 203, 206, 212, 213, 214, 229
Lessing, G. E., 185, 193, 196
Lévy, I., 76
Lienhard, M. K., 188
Lincoln, J. S., 36
Littré, E., 140, 146
Lommatzsch, E., xxii
Lucian, 98
Luther, W., 105
Lysias, 173

Malgaigne, J. F., 5
Malinowski, B., 38

Manrique, Jorge, 113
Marías, J., 120, 184
Marinus, 79
Mazon, P., 1
Menéndez Pelayo, M., 237
Méridier, L., 49, 111
Meseguer, P., 36
Metrodorus of Lampsacus, 10
Meuli, K., 42, 43, 74
Michel, C., 76, 77
Miller, A., 147
Miller, H. W., 216
Minturno, A. S., 185
Mireaux, E., 12
Moulinier, L., 2, 4, 17, 20, 41, 127, 129, 132
Müller, E., 187
Müri, W., 161
Murray, G., 2

Nestle, W., 33, 73, 74, 91, 92, 96, 97, 105, 140, 142, 145, 147, 164, 206, 216
Neuburger, M., 142
Newhall, S. N., 79
Nietzsche, F. W., 37, 55, 119, 204, 216, 219, 233, 236
Nilsson, M. P., 2, 8, 19, 20, 43, 44, 54, 56, 74, 76

Onians, R. B., 2, 12, 69
Oribasius, 60
Ortega y Gasset, J., 114, 214
Ovid, 60, 75

Pabón, J. M., 110
Pagel, J., 142
Palm, A., 36, 161
Papanoutsos, E. P., 188, 196
Parke, H. W., 41
Parmenides, 73, 80, 83, 89, 90, 92
Pauly, A., 26, 28, 127
Pausanias, 50, 53, 54, 55
Pazzini, A., 22
Peek, W., 65
Pericles, 32, 89
Pettenkofer, Max von, 3
Pfister, H. F., 21, 23, 26, 27, 28, 41, 50, 108, 127, 243

Index of Authors

Philodemus, 10
Philostratus, 98
Pindar, 38, 45, 46, 47, 51, 62, 63, 64, 66, 102, 105, 115, 217
Plato, 1, 4, 31, 35, 36, 38, 40, 42, 43, 44, 53, 57, 61, 67, 73, 78, 82, 86, 88, 91, 92, 100, 101, 105, 107, *108-38*, 139, 144, 156, 157, 158, 160, 164, 165, 166, 171, 172, 173, 174, 179, 188, 191, 192, 196, 206, 226, 238, 240, 241, 242, 243, 244, 245, 247
Plutarch, 104
Pohlenz, M., 194, 196, 198, 199, 200, 204
Porphyry, 78, 79
Preuss, K. T., 26
Proclus, 56, 79, 162, 187, 190
Prodicus, 104
Protagoras, 96, 102
Pseudo-Plutarch, 97, 98, 101
Pythagoras, 39, 42, 72, 74, 77, 78, 81, 82, 83, 86, 139

Rasch, W., 212
Rathmann, G., 76
Reitzenstein, R., 80
Renan, J. E., 9
Riess, 243
Rilke, R. M., 233
Robortello, F., 185
Rof Carballo, J., 41, 83
Rohde, E., 33, 40, 42, 54, 74, 76, 127, 190
Rose, V., 59, 73
Rostagni, A., 188, 196

Sappho, 64
Sartre, J. P., 216
Schadewaldt, W., *194-97*, 198, 200, 201, 203, 206, 208, 226, 233, 237
Scheftelowitz, I., 21, 27
Scheler, M., 212, 214
Schmiedeberg, O., 5
Schmitz, A., 107
Schottländer, R., 188
Schumacher, J., 81, 140, 142
Schwarz, O., 108

Scudéry, G. de, 185
Sellmair, J., 212
Sengle, F., 212, 214, 232, 238
Sigerist, H. E., 22, 25
Simonides of Ceos, 44
Snell, B., 9, 13, 14, 69, 114
Socrates, 31, 66, 67, 80, 93, 95, 97, 99, 100, 101, 111, 112, 113, 114, 115, 117, 122, 124, 125, 126, 129, 130, 136, 144, 165, 170, 183, 232, 237
Solmsen, F., 175
Solon, 20, 33, 34, 38, 89, 105, 216, 231
Sophocles, 38, 40, 47, 51, 54, 55, 63, 65, 67, 69, 70, 194, 206
Soranus, xxlii–xxiv
Stark, R., 188, 196, 238
Stengel, P., 19
Stenzel, J., 97, 104, 105
Stesichorus, 136
Suidas, 60, 98
Susemihl, F., 188
Süss, W., 105

Tamborino, J., 76, 77
Taylor, A. E., 149
Temkin, O., 141, 201, 202
Thales of Miletus, 14, 31, 72, 73, 87, 232
Theodorus, 173
Theognis, 33, 34, 35, 71, 72, 246
Theophrastus, 46, 220
Thespis, 232
Thrasymachus, 88, 112
Thucydides, 89, 207
Thurnwald, R., 22, 25
Tisias, 91, 172, 173
Tovar, A., 49, 53, 118, 173, 175
Tresmontant, C., 27
Tumarkin, A., 188

Ueberweg, F., 76, 83
Untersteiner, M., 105, 188, 238

Valera, J., 186
Valerius Flaccus, 127
Vedder, H., 10, 11
Veer, G. van der, 127

Index of Authors

Vegetius, xxi–xxii
Vergil, xxi
Virchow, R., 177
Volkmann-Schluck, K. H., 188, 196, 238

Wächter, T., 19
Walzel, O., 212
Weber, A., 212
Weil, H., 185, 187
Weinreich, O., 41
Weinstock, H., 188, 212, 216, 238
Welcker, F. G., 26, 33, 41, 108
Wellmann, M., 243

Wiedemann, K. A., 26
Wilamowitz, U. von, 60, 66, 79, 83, 203, 204, 205, 206, 228, 229
Wissowa, G., 21, 28, 127
Wormell, D. F. W., 41

Xenophanes, 72
Xenophon, 118, 122, 129, 206

Zafiropulo, J., 83
Zeller, E., 83
Zubiri, X., 11, 71, 74, 80, 87, 96, 205